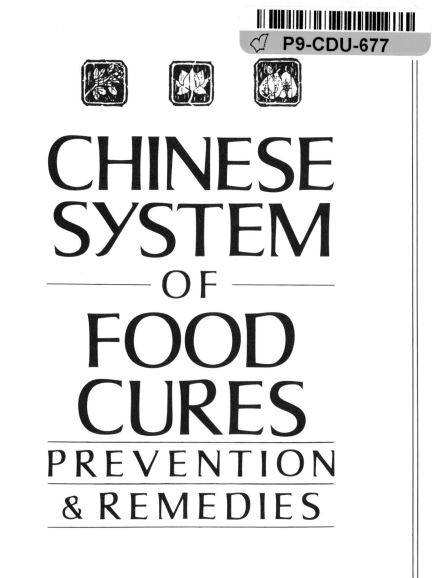

CHINESE SYSTEM

— OF —

FOOD CURES

PREVENTION
& REMEDIES

Henry C. Lu

 Sterling Publishing Co., Inc.   New York

P9-CDU-677

ACKNOWLEDGMENTS

I am greatly indebted to many professors of traditional Chinese medicine in China who allowed me to read their unpublished clinical reports and also to interview their patients, to many of my students who assisted me in the preparation of this manuscript, and also to many patients who discussed with me the treatment results of the formulas in this book. Their valuable contributions to this manuscript will always remain in my heart.

EDITED by VILMA LIACOURAS CHANTILES

Library of Congress Cataloging in Publication Data

Lu, Henry C.
  Chinese system of food cures.

  Bibliography: p.
  Includes index.
  1. Diet therapy. 2. Cookery, Chinese. 3. Medicine,
Chinese. I. Title.
RM216.L925 1986   615.8'54   86-5678
ISBN 0-8069-6308-5 (pbk.)

Contents

Foreword

I am delighted that Dr. Lu has written this excellent book about the Chinese system of food cures. It reflects not only his extensive clinical experience but also draws information from many Chinese diet classics as well as clinical reports and experiments conducted in China.

Chinese System of Food Cures: Prevention & Remedies presents to Western readers a completely new approach to the subject, although the Chinese people have practised it in China from time immemorial. The opening chapters, "Energies and Flavors of Foods" and "Actions of Food and the Balanced Diet," are truly remarkable; they introduce to the reader an entirely new concept of food and nutrition. "Body Types and the Yin-Yang Principles," the third chapter, offers insights into the principles of yin and yang and how they are traditionally applied to classify foods in relation to body types, moods, and the seasons. "Chinese Diet for Weight Loss" is a particularly fascinating chapter: It shows the reader how to lose weight effectively while enjoying foods and enhancing body energy.

All important aspects of foods are discussed in this book. In addition to their energies, flavors, and actions, the author includes practical food applications, clinical reports, and experiments, and adds many useful remarks on various aspects of foods. You should find "Preventing and Curing Ailments," the chapter dealing with treatments of common symptoms, very enlightening and beneficial. It covers a wide range of common ailments, such as coughing, hypertension, hiccupping, vomiting, diarrhea, stomachache, and others. Numerous foods and formulas for practical applications are listed under each symptom. Anyone with good health in mind will enjoy reading this chapter and will benefit from it.

In short, this is the freshest, most informative, and most useful book about food cures published in the English language.

WILLEM H. KHOE, M.D., D.Ac., D.Ht., D.Sc., Ph.D.

Introduction

The pioneer Chinese diet classic was published in 652 A.D. by Sun Shu Mao (581–682), a Chinese physician. He travelled with a bag of herbs and acupuncture gold needles, and is best remembered by the Chinese people as a roving herbalist and acupuncturist. He believed that a human life is more precious than one thousand ounces of gold, and for that reason, his book is entitled, *One Thousand Ounces of Gold Classic*.

In this classic, which contains thirty chapters, the dietary treatments of various diseases are discussed. Those for goitre, night blindness, and beriberi stand out as the most distinguished successes he achieved. Sun Shu Mao advanced the theory that goitre was caused by the patients' continual consumption of mountain water for a prolonged period of time. He then developed a dietary treatment of goitre using a formula of four essential ingredients— kelp, seaweed, and lamb and pork thyroid glands. He also introduced a treatment of night blindness by using beef, pork, and lamb livers. According to his theory, "the liver is associated with the eyes, and animal's liver can improve the conditions of human liver, which, in turn, contributes to the improvement of eyesight." This rationale is still applied in Chinese herbalism today. As for the dietary treatment of beriberi, his formula consisted of apricot seeds, cow's milk, and rice bran.

How can these three classic dietary formulas be evaluated by our modern medical knowledge? In the twentieth century we know that goitre is due to a lack of iodine in the diet and we also know that all the ingredients in Sun Shu Mao's formula for treatment of goitre are excellent sources of iodine. How about the formula for the treatment of night blindness? Our current medical knowledge indicates that night blindness results from vitamin A deficiency and that the livers of many animals are excellent sources of vitamin A. As for beriberi, the ingredients in Sun Shu Mao's formula are excellent sources of vitamin B-1 (thiamine), and beriberi is, according to modern medical science, due to lack of vitamin B-1 in the diet, usually a result of eating polished rice with the rice bran removed.

We still do not know everything about the causes and treatments of goitre, night blindness, and beriberi. Just look, for example, at the following quotations from the well-known *Taber's Cyclopedic Medical Dictionary* to realize that the causes and treatments of the three diseases remain unsolved. Goitre, this dictionary indicates, "may be due to lack of iodine in diet," and night blindness "may result from vitamin A deficiency or hereditary factors." The expression *may be* is instructive here, because it indicates that we still lack a complete understanding of the causes and treatment of such diseases as goitre and night blindess.

Three important questions should be asked: Is it true that goitre is caused by a lack of iodine alone, that night blindness is caused by vitamin A deficiency alone, and that beriberi is caused by vitamin B-1 deficiency alone? The Chinese physicians' answers to these questions are all negative, partly because the concepts of iodine and vitamins do not form part of traditional Chinese theory, and partly because many Chinese herbs used to treat goitre, night blindness, and beriberi do not contain iodine or vitamin A or vitamin B-1. I believe a few examples should illustrate this point very adequately.

• According to a clinical report written by the Chinese Pharmacological Research Institute of Jilin Province in China and published in *Chinese Herbs Reporter*, Volume No. 6 (1972), three herbal prescriptions in tablet form were used to treat goitre: The first prescription contained only willow leaves (salix babylonica L.), with each tablet weighing .5 g, which equalled 2 g dry willow leaves; the second prescription contained willow leaves and seaweed with each tablet weighing .5 g, which equalled 2 g dry willow leaves and .5 g dried seaweed; the third prescription contained willow leaves and two other herbs, yellow seeds (dioscorea bulbifera L.) and white seeds (stephnia cepharantha Hayata), with each tablet weighing .5 g, which equalled .6 g dried willow leaves and .65 g dried yellow seeds and .1 g dried white seeds. In the course of the treatment, adults took eight to ten tablets or as many as fifteen tablets each day, divided into three dosages for two months as one course of treatment; dosages were reduced for children. According to this report, the third prescription produced the best results: a 44.8 percent cure rate and 100 percent effective rate. According to modern Chinese research, 100 g dried willow leaves contain 1,500 to 2,500 mg iodine; in the second prescription, seaweed contains plenty of iodine, as commonly acknowledged in modern diet. But in the third prescription, the yellow seeds contain diosgenin and the white seeds contain trilobine but neither contains any iodine.

• In July 1984, I received a letter from my brother in Taiwan indicating that my niece was suffering from severe goitre and had to undergo an operation soon unless I could come up with some herbal remedy for her. Since the situation was very urgent, I immediately rushed the above third prescription to her by airmail. I was glad to receive my brother's letter three months later, disclosing that my niece had recovered from goitre. If my niece had only needed iodine, she would have got it locally instead of writing to me for help, which means that iodine itself is not as effective as the traditional Chinese herbal formula.

• Virtually all herbal formulas traditionally used to treat goitre in Chinese medicine include some ingredients with abundant iodine, notably seaweed, sea grass, and kelp; this is a fact. But at the same time, the formulas also include other ingredients with no iodine in them. These formulas, which have been developed on the basis of the traditional theory of Chinese medicine, are unintelligible from the viewpoint of Western medicine. And the same principle applies in the treatment of thyroid tumors. For example, according to a clinical report written by two Chinese doctors and published in *Fujian Medical Journal*, Volume No. 2 (1964), yellow seeds were used to treat 25 cases of thyroid tumor, which produced an 80 percent effective rate (20 cases) and 20 percent ineffective rate (five cases), compared to the ten cases in the control group treated with iodine, which produced a 20 percent effective rate (two cases) and 80 percent ineffective rate (eight cases).

• A Chinese herb, grey rhizome (atractylodes lancea Thunb. D.C.), has been traditionally used to treat night blindness. According to a report written by Dr. Ren-De Yeh published in *Canton Chinese Medical Journal*, Volume No. 1 (1960), five cases of night blindness were treated with this herb for two to three days and all were cured. Subsequent observations confirmed that the effects were permanent. The grey rhizome contains atractylol and hinesol, but it contains no vitamin A, which is now considered beneficial in curing night blindness.

• According to a clinical report prepared by the First Hospital in the city of Fuzhou, China, published in *Chinese Herbs Reporter*, Volume No. 3 (1971), of the 5,000 beriberi cases treated by a herbal formula in the past ten years, an effective rate higher than 90 percent was established. In light cases, it took only five to seven treatments, and in more severe cases two to three courses of treatments. This formula was found equally effective for both dry beriberi and wet beriberi; the formula contained only two ingredients, wild monkey persimmon (rosa bracteata Wendl.) and garlic stalk. Each dosage consisted of 10 g dried wild monkey persimmons and 15 g fresh garlic stalks (if garlic stalks were not available, 7 g garlic cloves were used). The ingredients were boiled in two cups water over low heat until the water was reduced to one cup, which was divided into two dosages, one for morning and one for evening. Each course of the treatment lasted from five to seven days, with two courses of treatment or longer as a program.

It is worth mentioning that wild monkey persimmon contains no vitamins and garlic clove contains about .24 mg vitamin B-1 per 100 g, which is comparatively less than pork kidney or chicken egg yolk. The same observation is clear as in the treatment of goitre: One ingredient contains vitamin B-1 (now considered beneficial for beriberi), but the other ingredient contains no vitamin B-1. Thus, from the viewpoint of Western medicine, there is one known factor and still an unknown factor involved in the traditional Chinese formulas for goitre and beriberi.

Perhaps the most revealing fact is that the dietary treatments discovered in China in the seventh century are still valid today. Western doctors in the seventh century would have been greatly puzzled by the Chinese methods of treating goitre, night blindness, beriberi, and other diseases, because on the one hand, they were not prepared to accept the traditional Chinese theory, and on the other, they lacked the knowledge about vitamins that explains the obviously successful treatment of these diseases by Chinese methods. Certainly a gap existed between Chinese and Western medicine. Unfortunately the same gap continues to exist. I wrote this book primarily to bridge the gap between East and West in the interest of human health.

Undoubtedly, in modern China, Chinese diet and herbs have been used with great success to treat many seemingly incurable diseases, including skin diseases, hepatitis, rheumatism, and even cancers. But these treatments have been ignored by the Western medical profession. The fact that Chinese diet and herbs work rather effectively means a great deal to the advancement of world medicine, despite Western medical scientists' unwillingness to investigate traditional Chinese medical theory. In medicine, as well as in other fields of inquiry, certainly there are always unknown factors. In the seventh century, Western medical scientists did not know that kelp and seaweed could be used to treat goitre because of the iodine content, or that animals' liver could be used to treat night blindness because of the vitamin A content, or that rice bran could be used to treat beriberi because of the vitamin B-1 content, but they are now aware of these facts.

In other words, the unknown factors in the seventh century about the Chinese treatment of goitre by kelp and seaweed, of night blindness by liver, or of beriberi by rice bran have become the *known* factors. Over the years, countless classics have been published in which Chinese doctors continued to develop more effective methods of medical treatment. The unknown factors must have proportionally increased for Western medical scientists. And it is certainly unscientific to disregard any successful medical treatments because of unknown factors. Can we say that a patient is not really ill just because we cannot diagnose the disease? Can we disregard an obviously successful treatment because we do not know how it works?

I believe that modern Western medical scientists should try to explore the unknown factors in Chinese medical approaches to human health instead of avoiding them. Then the unknown factors may become the known factors— a true measure of human progress. This book is dedicated to that objective.

Henry C. Lu
Vancouver, British Columbia, Canada

Before You Begin

You may wonder how to prepare and store food cures and what to expect when you begin taking them. The important thing is to be persistent. Food cures show results only after a relatively long period, ranging from one week to a few months or even longer. You may want to continue a cure throughout your life if it has proven beneficial to your health. For example, if you suffer from chronic constipation, you may drink one to two glasses of milk on an empty stomach every morning for months or years, or take one or two teaspoonfuls of honey dissolved in warm water (also on an empty stomach) for as long as you please.

Sometimes you may have to quit for a while. Suppose you are treating hemorrhoids, but in the middle of using food cures, you catch a cold and develop a fever. You may have to interrupt your food cures of hemorrhoids and start drinking one or two glasses of fresh ginger soup to cope with your common cold. After you have recovered from the cold, you can start the program of food cures for hemorrhoids all over again. Another example is that your symptoms may very often, but by no means always, be consistent with your physical type. Suppose you have a yang physical type; yin foods are normally good for you. But if you suddenly develop cold stomachache (a yin symptom), then yang foods are better for you than yin foods because they can help eliminate your symptoms. Generally speaking, however, the disease you suffer from will be consistent with your physical type.

MAKING AND STORING THE FOOD CURES

The preparation of Chinese food cures is not the same as general Chinese cooking. Unless it is specified, when making food cures and remedies in this book, no oil is used. In everyday cookery, "fry" usually means to fry in a large quantity of oil, and sauté or stir-fry means to use a small quantity of oil or fat. In this book, the verb "fry" means to fry *without* oil. It is more like toasting a food in a pan, allowing the heat to penetrate the food to toast the surface.

A very important way of frying foods for cures is to fry them without oil until the surface appears brown, yellowish, or close to black while the interior remains the same as it was. This method is used mostly for grinding the foods into powder; there are many variations of preparing foods for this purpose. Traditionally, the Chinese wrapped the foods in a wet cloth and put the wrapped foods in among burning charcoals; but now we can use aluminum foil to wrap foods. We can also dry foods over low heat or bake or roast them; but always make certain that the foods are equally or almost equally dry inside and outside, which is called "drying the foods by fire while retaining their original nature" in the Chinese system of food cures.

Other cookery terms and methods are more familiar to both Chinese and Western readers: When a food is boiled, it is boiled in water, unless specified otherwise. Often the food or herb is strained and only the broth or liquid is consumed as soup or tea. For other remedies, after cooking the food in water, you may eat the food and drink the liquid as the recipe suggests.

The foods used for food cures are generally not kept for very long, except in powdered form. But even powder should be stored in the refrigerator. Make certain that the powder is really dry when you grind it.

As for the amounts, use common sense when following the suggestions in the subsequent chapters. It is important to emphasize that quantities given with each food are *approximate* only. You can make adjustments to meet your own needs. A person can eat one banana a day or three bananas a day for the hemorrhoid or constipation cures, which should not make a significant difference when recommending foods, not herbs or drugs.

When spoonfuls are suggested in this book, they always mean teaspoonfuls, unless otherwise specified. Other measurements and equivalents can be adjusted by referring to the Conversion Guides.

SPECIAL PREPARATIONS

Rice wine, rice vinegar, fresh ginger juice, salt and honey are the five ingredients you can use to prepare foods to your specifications.

• *Rice wine:* In this book, always use rice wine when the recipe calls for wine. There are three ways you can use rice wine to prepare foods: (1) While you are frying food, add wine in the process until it is dry; the quantity of wine may be individually adjusted. (2) Soak foods in wine for a few hours before frying. (3) When boiling foods, add some wine before removing from the heat. The purpose of using wine to prepare foods is to make them move upwards, which is good for symptoms in the upper body region, such as headache with a common cold.

• *Rice vinegar:* Use rice vinegar the same way as rice wine but for a different purpose. Rice vinegar is normally used to increase the constrictive effects of foods, which is particularly useful in curing diarrhea and stopping bleeding.

• *Fresh ginger juice:* (1) Fresh ginger juice may be added to soup before it is removed from the heat. (2) Foods may be cooked with a suitable amount of fresh ginger soup. The purpose of preparing foods with fresh ginger soup is to increase their yang nature so that the foods will move outward and become more effective for cold symptoms.

• *Salt:* Place an adequate amount of salt in a glass of water and stir it until completely dissolved; then pour the salt water into the pan while cooking the food; continue cooking until the water evaporates and the food becomes yellowish. The purpose of using salt to prepare foods is to make food move downwards—good for abdominal pain and constipation.

• *Honey:* Place a few tablespoonfuls of honey in the pan and heat it over low heat until honey becomes yellowish; add water and stir it. Then add the food and cook together until a little dry and very difficult to separate by hand. The purpose of preparing food with honey is to increase the degree of lubrication of the food, which is very desirable for curing a cough.

Conversion Guides

CUSTOMARY TERMS		METRIC SYMBOLS	
t.	teaspoon	ml or mL	millilitre
T.	tablespoon	L	litre
c.	cup	mg	milligram
pkg.	package	g	gram
pt.	pint	kg	kilogram
qt.	quart	mm	millimetre
oz.	ounce	cm	centimetre
lb.	pound	°C	degrees Celsius
°F	degrees Fahrenheit		
in.	inch		

Guide to Approximate Equivalents

CUSTOMARY					METRIC
Ounces Pounds	Cups	Tablespoons	Teaspoons	Millilitres	Grams Kilograms
			¼ t.	1 ml	1g
			½ t.	2 ml	
			1 t.	5 ml	
			2 t.	10 ml	
½ oz.		1 T.	3 t.	15 ml	15 g
1 oz.		2 T.	6 t.	30 ml	28 g
2 oz.	¼ c.	4 T.	12 t.	60 ml	60 g
4 oz.	½ c.	8 T.	24 t.	125 ml	120 g
8 oz.	1 c.	16 T.	48 t.	250 ml	225 g
1 lb.					450 g
	4 c.			1 L	
2.2 lb.					1 kg

Keep in mind that this is not an exact conversion, but generally may be used for food measurement.

Equivalent Food and Cookery Terms

American	British	American	British
All-purpose flour	Plain flour	Ground meat	Minced meat
Bacon	Rashers	ground (spice)	(spice) powder
Broil	Grill	Heavy cream	Double cream
Brown sugar	Demerara sugar	Light cream	Single cream
Candy	Sweets; confections	Molasses	Treacle
Confectioners' sugar	Icing sugar	Rock candy	Rock sugar
Cookie	Biscuit	Scallion	Spring or green onion
Cornstarch	Cornflour	Shrimp	Prawn
Eggplant	Aubergine	Squid (calamari)	Inkfish
Strain	Filter	Zucchini	Baby marrow or
Fine granulated white sugar	Caster (castor) sugar		courgette

1
Energies and Flavors of Foods

THE CHINESE DIET: DIFFERENCES FROM WESTERN DIET

There are two basic differences between Chinese and Western diets. First of all, Western diet focuses almost exclusively on diet for weight loss. Chinese diet is designed not only to help you lose weight but also to treat many other ailments, including hypertension, diabetes, common cold, gastritis, diarrhea, constipation, cough, hepatitis, psoriasis, common acne, eczema, and so on.

In Chinese diet, for example, it is considered bad for someone with constipation to drink tea; it is good for someone with a cough to eat apple with honey. When I have a headache, I want to know which foods I should eat to cure my headache and which I should avoid to prevent my headache from becoming worse. When I have diarrhea or am suffering from diabetes, I want to know which foods I should eat to treat my symptoms, and which to avoid to prevent my problems from becoming worse. When I am overweight, I want to know which foods I should eat to reduce my weight and which not to eat to avoid gaining more weight.

To lose weight, no doubt, is part of Chinese diet, but there are many other considerations as important as weight loss in the minds of Chinese dietitians. Recently, I read a diet book written by a well-known Western physician, and to my great amazement, I found no information on dietary treatment of such symptoms as sore throat, hemorrhoids, hiccupping, vomiting, fever, toothache, psoriasis, stomachache, and other ailments—all important treatments when using the Chinese diet.

The second difference between Chinese and Western diets: In Western diet, foods are considered for their protein, calorie, carbohydrate, vitamin, and other nutrient content, but in Chinese diet, foods are considered for their flavors, energies, movements, and common and organic actions. It works like this: If I feel cold in my body and limbs, naturally I like to eat something that will warm me; if I feel hot, something to cool me. If I have a weak stomach, naturally I like to eat something that will make my stomach stronger; if I feel my kidneys are weakening, something that will make my kidneys stronger. Ginger will warm me, because it has a warm energy; mung beans will cool me, because they have a cool energy; sugar can make my stomach stronger, because it tastes sweet and acts on the stomach; yam will make my kidneys stronger, because it acts on the kidneys in a special way.

To be sure, we can find nutritional information on foods in Western diet. For example, we know that red pepper contains vitamins A and C, but it does not tell us that it can warm us; we know mung beans contain some protein and carbohydrates, but not that mung beans can cool us; we know that black pepper contains some protein, but not that it can make our stomachs stronger; we know that yam contains protein, carbohydrate, calcium, and many vitamins, but not that it can make our kidneys stronger. Thus, it is easy to see how Chinese diet differs from Western diet.

The essential aspects of Chinese diet in regard to foods are: the five flavors of foods, the five energies of foods, the movements of foods, and the common and organic actions of foods.

THE FIVE FLAVORS OF FOODS

The five flavors of foods include pungent (acrid), sweet, sour, bitter, and salty.

Pungent foods include green onion, chive, clove, parsley, and coriander.

Sweet foods include sugar, cherry, chestnut, and banana.

Sour foods include lemon, pear, plum, and mango.

Bitter foods include hops, lettuce, radish leaf, and vinegar (I list vinegar as bitter because the Chinese call vinegar "bitter wine." Vinegar tastes both sour and bitter; it is common for some foods to have two simultaneous flavors).

Salty foods include salt, kelp, and seaweed.

The flavors of foods are important in Chinese diet, because different flavors have their respective important effects upon the internal organs. Foods that have a pungent flavor can act on the lungs and large intestine; foods with a sweet flavor on the stomach and spleen; with sour flavor on the liver and gall bladder; with a bitter flavor on the heart and small intestine; foods that have a salty flavor can act on the kidneys and bladder.

Let's take the sweet flavor as an example, that acts on the stomach and spleen. It is common knowledge among Chinese and Western dietitians, that eating sweet foods will put on weight, but Chinese and Western dietitians give different explanations. According to Western dietitians, eating sweet foods puts on weight because sweet foods contain a large number of calories; according to Chinese dietitians, eating sweet foods will put on weight because sweet foods can act on the stomach and spleen, which are in charge of digestive functions. In other words, in Chinese diet, sweet foods are considered capable of improving the digestive functions, which is why they are good for people with a weak digestive system. In talking to a Western audience about Chinese diet, one question frequently comes up: How do we determine the flavors of such foods as beef, pork, and celery that have no distinct tastes? In Chinese diet, beef has a sweet flavor, pork has a sweet and salty flavor, and celery a sweet flavor. Some foods have one flavor, but others may have two or three. Undoubtedly, the flavors of many foods are very difficult to determine precisely, but the Chinese have done it through many centuries of experience.

The process may look like this: At the beginning, some foods with obvious flavors are found to act on some internal organs and perform specific actions in the human body. The basic relationships between flavors and internal organs and the actions are studied and analyzed by a process in science called the inductive method. As time goes on, other foods whose flavors are more difficult to determine may be found capable of acting upon some internal organs and performing some specific actions. The flavors of such foods are determined on the basis of their organic effects and specific actions. This process in science is called the deductive method.

In general, the common actions of foods in regard to their flavors are as follows:

Pungent foods (ginger, green onion, and peppermint) can induce perspiration and promote energy circulation.

Sweet foods (honey, sugar, and watermelon) can slow down the acute symptoms and neutralize the toxic effects of other foods.

Sour foods (lemon and plum) can obstruct the movements, and are useful, therefore, in checking diarrhea and excessive perspiration.

Bitter foods, such as animals' gall bladder and hops, can reduce body heat, dry body fluids, and induce diarrhea (which is why many Chinese herbs recommended to reduce fever and induce diarrhea taste bitter).

Salty foods (kelp and seaweed) can soften hardness, which explains their usefulness in treating tuberculosis of the lymph nodes and other symptoms involving the hardening of muscles or glands.

In addition, some foods have a light flavor or little taste. These foods normally have two flavor classifications. Cucumber, for example, has sweet and light flavors. Foods with a light flavor promote urination and may be used as diuretics. Job's tears is one of the outstanding examples.

The following are foods arranged by different flavors:

• *Bitter*: apricot seed, asparagus, bitter gourd, wild cucumber, celery, cherry seed, coffee, grapefruit peel, hops, kohlrabi, lettuce, lotus plumule, radish leaf, sea grass, vinegar, wine.

• *Slightly bitter*: ginseng, pumpkin.

• *Light*: Job's tears, kidney bean, sunflower seed, white fungus, Chinese wax gourd.

• *Pungent*: black pepper, castor bean, cherry seed, chive, chive root, chive seed, cinnamon bark, cinnamon twig, clove, Chinese parsley, cottonseed, dillseeds, fennel, garlic, ginger, dried or fresh, grapefruit peel, green onion, leaf and white head, green pepper, kohlrabi, kumquat, leaf mustard, leek, marjoram, nutmeg, peppermint, radish and radish leaf, red pepper, rice bran, rosemary, soybean oil, spearmint, star anise, sweet basil, taro, tobacco, white pepper, wine.

• *Slightly pungent*: asparagus, caraway.

• *Salty*: abalone, barley, chive seeds, clam (sea, fresh water, river clamshell, sea clamshell), crab, cuttlebone, cuttlefish, duck, eel blood, ham, kelp, milk (human), oyster, oyster shell, pork, salt, seagrass, seaweed. (All recommended shells are crushed into powder before using them.)

• *Sour*: apple, apricot, crab apple, grape, grapefruit, hawthorn fruits, kumquat, litchi, loquat, mandarin orange, mango, olive, peach, pineapple, plum, raspberry, small red or adzuki bean, star fruit or carambola, strawberry, tangerine, tomato, vinegar.

• *Extremely sour*: lemon, pear, sour plum.

• *Sweet*: abalone, apple, apricot, apricot seeds (sweet), bamboo shoots, banana, barley, bean curd, beef, beetroots, black fungus, black sesame seeds, black soybean, brown sugar, cabbage (Chinese), carp (common carp, gold carp, grass carp), carrot, castor bean, celery, cherry, chestnut, chicken, chicken egg, yolk and white, Chinese wax gourd, cinnamon bark, cinnamon twig, clam (fresh water), coconut, coffee, common button mushroom, corn, corn silk, crab apple, cucumber, red and black date, dry mandarin orange peel, duck, eel, eel blood, eggplant, fig, ginseng, grape, grapefruit, grapefruit peel, guava, guava leaf, hawthorn fruits, honey, horse bean, hyacinth bean, Job's tears, kidney bean, kohlrabi, kumquat, lettuce, licorice, lily flower, litchi, longan, longevity fruit, loquat, lotus (fruit and seed), malt, maltose, mandarin orange, mango, milk (cow's and human), mung bean, muskmelon, mutton, olive, oyster, papaya, peach, peanuts, pear, persimmon, pineapple, plum, pork, potato, pumpkin, radish, raspberry, red small bean or adzuki bean, rice bran, rice (polished), saffron, sesame oil, shiitake mushroom, shrimp, soybean oil, spearmint, spinach, squash, star anise, star fruit, strawberry, string bean, sugar cane, sunflower seed, sweet rice, sweet potato, sword bean, tangerine-orange, taro, tomato, walnut, water chestnut, watermelon, wheat, wheat bran, white fungus, white sugar, wine, yellow soybean.

THE FIVE ENERGIES OF FOODS

The energies of foods refer to their capacity to generate sensations—either hot or cold—in the human body. As an example, eating foods with a hot energy will make us experience hot sensations in the body, and foods with a cold energy, cold sensations. In daily life, each of us knows that eating ice makes us feel cold and drinking hot water makes us feel warm. This is because ice has a cold energy and hot water, a hot energy. But ice or hot water produce only temporary effects. To produce longlasting effects, herbs are used as substitutes for foods that provide only temporary relief. In other words, to produce cold or hot sensations, herbs are more effective than foods, and foods are more effective than ice or hot water.

The five energies of foods are cold, hot, warm, cool, and neutral. But the adjectives, "cold," "hot," "warm," "cool," "neutral," do not refer to the *present* state of foods. For example, tea has a cold energy, so even though you may drink hot tea, you are actually drinking a cold beverage. Shortly after the tea enters your body, its heat (a temporary phenomenon) will be lost and as it begins to generate cold energy, your body begins to cool off. Another example, red pepper has a hot energy. Even though you may eat *cold* red pepper from the refrigerator, you still consume a hot food. Shortly after it enters your body, its temporary coldness is lost, and your body begins to feel hot.

When I discuss the energies of foods, therefore, I refer to what the foods do in our bodies—*whether they generate hot or cold, warm or cool, or neutral sensations.* Hot is opposed to cold; warm is opposed to cool; neutral is somewhere between warm and cool. Cold and cool foods differ from each other, as do warm and hot foods. Bamboo shoots have a cold energy, black pepper a hot energy; cucumber has a cool energy, chicken a warm, and corn a neutral energy.

It is important for us to know the energies of foods, because different energies act upon the human body in different ways. This has important effects on good health. As an example, when a person suffers from cold rheumatism and the pain is particularly severe on cold winter days, then it is good for him or her to eat foods with a warm or hot energy, which should considerably relieve the pain. Or if you suffer from skin eruptions that worsen when exposed to heat, it is good to eat foods with a cold or cool energy to relieve your symptoms.

While the energies of foods play an important role in Chinese diet, the Chinese also classify the human body into cold and hot types. One person may have a hot physical constitution, another a cold one. The person with a hot physical constitution should consume more foods with a cold or cool energy; the person with a cold physical constitution, more foods with a hot or warm energy—a plan the Chinese call "a balanced diet." Such a diet is always related to each individual's physical constitution and may differ from one person to another.

During my lectures and in my clinical practice, people often ask me: Is tea good? Is coffee better than tea? Is liquor good for you? There are no absolute answers. In fact, these are the wrong questions. It would make more sense to ask: Is tea good for me? Which is better for me, coffee or tea? Is it good for me to drink liquor? Those questions can be answered correctly. Tea is good for you if you have a hot physical constitution, because tea has a cold energy; if you have a cold physical constitution, coffee is better for you than tea, because coffee has a warm energy. If you have a cold physical constitution, liquor can warm you, but if you have a hot physical constitution, it may create many symptoms of certain hot diseases, such as skin problems. For this reason, in the Chinese diet, foods with a cold energy are used to counteract intoxication and alcoholism.

The process of learning the energies of foods is basically the same as that of finding the flavors of foods. At first, the foods that *obviously* make us feel hot may be considered as having a hot energy; the foods that make us cold, a cold energy. For example, obviously ice makes us feel cold, so it is believed to have a cold energy; and since red pepper makes us feel hot, it is thought to have a hot energy. As time goes on, *any* food that can make us hot is regarded as having a hot energy; any food that can make us cold, a cold energy.

It's interesting to see how important and relevant the energies of foods in Chinese diet can be. Suppose on a cold rainy day, on your way home from work, your car breaks down. You walk to a service station to hire a tow truck and by the time you get home, you're soaked to the skin and shivering with cold. You suspect that you caught cold. If you have some knowledge of the Chinese diet, you prepare a bowl of fresh old ginger soup and drink it hot. You feel much better, because fresh old ginger has a warm energy that warms you, and a pungent flavor that makes you perspire.

Let's use another example. Suppose you develop hives with severe itching. You cannot cook your meals, because the heat in the kitchen makes your itching intolerable. If you have a fair knowledge about Chinese diet, you cook a bowl of mung bean soup and stir in some sugar. After drinking the soup a few times, your symptoms disappear, because the cold energy in both mung beans and sugar heal your hot symptoms. Of course, many other factors need to be considered as well, but the energy of foods is important.

Suppose you suffer from hemorrhoids and know about Chinese diet. You eat two cooked (underdone) whole bananas (*with the peels*) every day. The bananas should improve the symptoms, because banana has a cold energy.

On the negative side, let's suppose you have no knowledge about Chinese diet and you happen to make a mistake. In the first example, when you had the cold, instead of drinking hot ginger soup, you drank a bowl of mung bean soup. That would have made your symptoms worse. With the hives, had you taken hot sauce at dinner instead of mung bean soup, your itching would probably have become much worse. With the hemorrhoids, if instead of eating bananas, you drank whiskey every day, that too could make your symptoms deteriorate.

The following foods arranged by their different energies:
• *Cold*: bamboo shoot, banana, bitter gourd, clam (sea and freshwater), clam-

shell, crab, grapefruit, kelp, lettuce, lotus plumule, muskmelon, persimmon, salt, sea grass, seaweed, star fruit, sugar cane, water chestnut, watermelon.
• *Slightly cold*: hops, tomato.
• *Cool energy*: apple, barley, bean curd, chicken egg white, Chinese wax gourd, common button mushroom, cucumber, eggplant, Job's tears, lettuce, lily flower, longevity fruit, loquat, mandarin orange, mango, marjoram, mung bean, oyster shell, pear, peppermint, radish, sesame oil, spinach, strawberry; tangerine, wheat, wheat bran.
• *Hot*: black pepper, cinnamon bark, cottonseed, ginger (dried ginger), green pepper, red pepper, soybean oil, white pepper.
• *Neutral*: abalone, apricot, beef, beetroot, black fungus, black sesame seed, black soybean, cabbage (Chinese), carp (common carp, gold carp), carrot, castor bean, celery, cherry seed, chicken egg, chicken egg yolk, corn, corn silk, crab apple, cuttlefish, dry mandarin orange peel, duck, eel blood, fig, grape, guava leaf, honey, horse bean, hyacinth bean, kidney bean, kohlrabi, licorice, lotus fruit and seed, milk (cow's and human), olive, oyster, papaya, peanuts, pineapple, plum, polished rice, pork, potato, pumpkin, radish leaf, small red or adzuki bean, rice bran, saffron, shiitake mushroom, sour plum, string bean, sunflower seed, sweet rice, sweet potato, taro, taro flower, white fungus, white sugar, yellow soybean.
• *Warm*: apricot seed (bitter and sweet apricot), brown sugar, caraway, carp (grass carp), cherry, chestnut, chicken, chive, chive seeds, chive roots, cinnamon twig, clove, coconut, coffee, coriander (Chinese parsley), date (both red and black), dillseeds, eel, fennel, garlic, ginger (fresh ginger), ginseng, grapefruit peel, green onion leaf, green onion white head, guava, ham, kumquat, leaf mustard, leek, litchi, longan, maltose, mutton, nutmeg, peach, raspberry, rosemary, shrimp, spearmint, squash, star anise, sunflower seed, sweet basil, sword bean, tobacco, vinegar, walnut, wine.
• *Slightly warm*: asparagus, cuttlebone, hawthorn fruits, malt.

THE MOVEMENTS OF FOODS

Foods have a tendency to move in different directions in the body. Some foods move outward, some inward; some foods have a tendency to move upwards; some downwards. To see how this works, think of the human body as divided into four regions: inside (internal region); outside (skin and body surface); upper (above the waist); lower (below the waist).

To move outward means to move from inside towards outside; so foods with outward movements can induce perspiration and reduce fever.

To move inward means to move from outside towards inside; so foods with inward movements can ease bowel movements and abdominal swelling.

To move upwards means to move from the lower region towards the upper region; so foods with upward movements can relieve diarrhea, prolapse of anus, prolapse of uterus, and falling of stomach.

To move downwards means to move from the upper region towards the lower region; so foods with downward movements can relieve vomiting, hiccupping, and asthma.

In general, leaves and flowers have a tendency to move upwards. Roots and seeds and fruits have a tendency to move downwards. But this is just a general principle. There are many exceptions.

Among the foods we eat every day, peppermint has a tendency to move outward; banana has a tendency to move inward; wine has a tendency to move upwards; salt has a tendency to move downwards. Some foods can move in two directions.

Two additional characteristics of food are associated with the movements, namely, glossy (sliding) and obstructive. Glossy foods, such as honey and spinach, facilitate the movements. Obstructive foods, such as guava and olive, slow down the movements. Glossy foods are good for constipation and internal dryness, but bad for diarrhea and seminal emission. Conversely, obstructive foods are good for diarrhea and seminal emission, but bad for constipation and internal dryness. The movements of foods are important in Chinese diet, because foods moving in different directions have different applications in coping with human health problems.

The symptoms treated by the different movements of foods are classified into four categories: First, upward symptoms, such as vomiting, hiccupping, coughing, etc., should be treated by foods that can move downwards. Second, downward symptoms, such as diarrhea, falling of the stomach, and prolapse of uterus and anus, should be treated by foods that can move upwards. Third, the outward symptoms, such as excessive perspiration, premature ejaculation, seminal emission, frequent urination, shoud be treated by foods that can obstruct. The inward symptoms, such as constipation and abdominal swelling, should be treated by foods that can move outward in combination with other foods that cleanse the internal regions.

The movements of foods change after they are prepared in a certain way. Foods prepared with wine develop a tendency to move upwards. That is the reason, in treating falling symptoms like prolapse of uterus and anus, herbs are very often processed along with the wine. Foods prepared with ginger juice develop a tendency to move outward. When foods are prepared with vinegar, they have a tendency to become obstructive. Foods processed with salt (as in frying) develop a tendency to move downwards.

In clinical practice, we often see patients with falling of the stomach, which is called gastroptosis in Western medicine. When a patient with this symptom consults a physician, he or she is often told to stay upside down so that the stomach is restored to its original position. This sounds like a sensible treatment, because when the person is upside down, the stomach will surely fall in the opposite direction—but it's impractical. A person is born to stand on his feet and not on his head. And it is also ineffective, because when the person stands upright, the stomach will fall again.

From the Chinese point of view, a far more effective treatment of this downward symptom is to eat foods that can move upwards, so they will push up the energy. Although none of the common foods we eat every day push upwards forcefully, plenty of herbs do the job very effectively. For example, *rhizoma cimicifugae* is called the "elevating herb" because of its power to push upwards. *Radix bupleuri* is also used for the same purpose.

The movements of foods are also related to the flavors and energies of foods. Generally, warm and hot foods that have a pungent and sweet flavor tend to move upwards or outward; cold and cool foods that have a sour or salty or bitter flavor tend to move downwards or inward. In addition, the movements of foods also relate to the four seasons: Foods that move upwards are good to consume in spring, the time when living things begin to grow; growth means to move upwards. Foods that move outward are good in summer, when everything is outgoing (as in perspiration and expansion). Foods that move downwards are good in autumn, when things begin to fall (such as leaves). Foods that move inward are good in winter, when things move inward (and stay indoors). The following foods are arranged by their combinations of energies and flavors suitable for the four seasons.

• Foods with an *upward movement* are good to eat in *spring*. Such foods have a neutral energy and three flavors—pungent or sweet or bitter. These include abalone, apricot, beef, beetroots, black fungus, black sesame seed, black soybean, cabbage (Chinese), carp (common and gold carp), carrot, celery, cherry seed, chicken egg, chicken egg yolk, corn silk, crab apple, dry mandarin orange peel, duck, eel blood, fig, grape, guava leaf, honey, horse bean, hyacinth bean, kidney bean, kohlrabi, licorice, lotus fruit and seed, milk (cow's and human milk), olive, oyster, peanuts, pineapple, plum, pork, potato, pumpkin, radish leaf, small red bean or adzuki bean, rice bran, saffron, shiitake mushroom, string bean, sunflower seed, sweet rice, sweet potato, taro, white fungus, white sugar, yellow soybean.

Foods with an *outward movement* are good in *summer*. These foods have a hot energy and two different flavors—pungent or sweet. Among these are black pepper, cinnamon bark, cottonseed, ginger (dried), green pepper; red pepper; soybean oil; white pepper.

Foods with a *downward movement*, good in *autumn*. Such foods have three energies—cold or cool or warm—and two flavors—sweet or sour. This list includes apple, bamboo shoots, banana, barley, bean curd, chicken egg white, Chinese wax gourd, clam (freshwater), common button mushroom, cucumber, eggplant, grapefruits, hawthorn fruits, kumquat, Job's tears, lettuce, lily flower, litchi, longevity fruit, loquat, mango, mung bean, muskmelon, peach, persimmon, spinach, star fruit, strawberry, sugar cane juice, tangerine, water chestnut, watermelon, wheat, wheat bran.

Foods with an *inward movement*, good in *winter*. They have a cold energy and two different flavors—bitter or salty. Bitter gourd, clam (salt and freshwater), crab, hops, kelp, lettuce, lotus plumule, salt, sea grass, and seaweed are among these foods.

2
Actions of Foods and the Balanced Diet

THE ORGANIC ACTIONS OF FOODS

Organic actions of foods refer to specific internal organs on which the foods can act. The Chinese people focus on ten internal organs for dietary treatment: lungs, large intestine, small intestine, gall bladder, bladder, liver, kidneys, spleen, heart, and stomach. Each food acts on one or more internal organs— the organic actions of that particular food. For example, celery acts on the stomach and liver, carrot on the lungs and spleen, eggplant on the spleen, stomach, and large intestine, wheat on the heart, spleen, and kidneys.

Flavors and energies of foods are important factors in determining the organic actions of foods. Generally, when the energy and flavor of a specific food are relatively simple, that food may only act on one organ. For example, almond is neutral and sweet, so it only acts on the lungs; wheat bran is cool and sweet, so it only acts on the stomach; kelp is cold and salty, so it only acts on the stomach. But when a food has more than one energy or one flavor, it may act on two or more organs at the same time. For example, tea is cool (or slightly cold) and bittersweet; it acts upon three internal organs—the heart, lungs, and stomach; barley is cool and sweet and salty; it acts on the spleen and stomach. But this is just a general principle, because many foods that have one energy and one flavor still act upon two or more internal organs simultaneously; and conversely, many foods that have two or more energies and flavors act only on one organ.

The organic actions of foods, like the flavors and energies of foods, have been discovered by the inductive and deductive methods throughout Chinese history. At first, certain foods may be effective in the treatment of some organic diseases. Consequently, such foods are considered good for specific actions on the diseased organs. This is arrived at by the inductive method. After many isolated instances have been observed, gradually, the results are used

23

to establish the associations between foods and internal organs. Chinese physicians have always put great emphasis on the relationships between internal organs and body surface, including the skin, the five senses, and visible symptoms. The diseases on body surface are then traced back to the related internal organs.

In Chinese belief, the eyes are associated with the liver; eye diseases may be traced to the liver. Ears are associated with the kidneys; deafness and hearing loss may be traced to the kidneys. The nose is associated with the lungs; disease of the nose may be traced to the lungs. Mouth and lips are associated with the spleen; mouth and lip diseases may be traced to the spleen. And since the tongue is associated with the heart, diseases of the tongue may be traced to the heart.

After the associations between internal organs and body surface are established, some foods may be found very effective when treating symptoms on the body surface. Gradually, these foods are used to establish the associations between foods and internal organs. This is arrived at by the deductive method. Chicken liver, for example, is effective for blurred vision; since the eyes are associated with the liver, it follows that the relationship between chicken liver and our liver may be established. Another example, honey is effective for relief of constipation—a symptom related to the large intestine—so that the association between honey and the large intestine is established. The following foods of different organic actions are listed with the organ on which they act.

• *Bladder*: Chinese wax gourd, cinnamon bark, cinnamon twig, fennel, grapefruit peel, watermelon.
• *Gall bladder*: chicory, corn silk.
• *Heart*: bitter gourd, chicken egg yolk, cinnamon twig, crab apple, green pepper, longan, lotus fruit and seed, lotus plumule, milk (cow's and human), mung bean, muskmelon, persimmon, red pepper, small red or adzuki bean, saffron, watermelon, wheat, wine.
• *Kidneys*: black sesame seed, black soybean, caraway, carp (common), chestnut, chicken egg yolk, chive, chive seeds, cinnamon bark, clam (freshwater), clove, cuttlebone, cuttlefish, dillseed, duck, eel, eel blood, fennel, grape, grapefruit peel, Job's tears, lotus fruit and seed, lotus plumule, mutton, oyster shell, plum, pork, salt, star anise, string bean, tangerine, walnut, wheat.
• *Large intestine*: bean curd, black fungus, black pepper, cabbage (Chinese), carp (gold carp), castor bean, Chinese wax gourd, corn, cucumber, eggplant, fig, honey, lettuce, nutmeg, persimmon, rice bran, salt, spinach, sweet basil, sword bean, taro, white pepper, yellow soybean.
• *Liver*: black sesame seed, brown sugar, celery, chicory, chive, chive seed, clam (freshwater), clamshell (river), corn silk, crab, crab apple, cuttlefish, eel, eel blood, hawthorn fruits, leek, litchi, loquat, oyster shell, peppermint, plum, saffron, sour plum, star anise, vinegar, wine.

• *Lungs*: carrot, castor bean, Chinese wax gourd, cinnamon twig, clamshell (river), common button mushroom, coriander, crab apple, duck, garlic, ginger (fresh and dried), ginseng, grape, green onion white head, honey, Job's tears, leaf mustard, leek, licorice, lily flower, loquat, lotus plumule, maltose, milk (cow's and human), olive, peanut, pear, peppermint, persimmon, radish, sugar cane, sweet basil, tangerine, walnut, water chestnut, wine.

• *Small intestine*: Chinese wax gourd, small red or adzuki bean, salt, spinach.

• *Spleen*: barley, bean curd, beef, bitter gourd, black soybean, brown sugar, carp (common, gold and grass), carrot, chestnut, chicken, cinnamon bark, clove, coriander, cucumber, date (red and black), dillseed, eel, eggplant, fig, garlic, ginger (fresh and dried), ginseng, grape, grapefruit peel, green pepper, hawthorn fruit, honey, horse bean, hyacinth bean, Job's tears, licorice, litchi, longan, loquat, lotus fruit and seed, malt, maltose, mutton, nutmeg, peanuts, pork, radish leaf, red pepper, rice (polished), squash, star anise, string bean, sweet basil, sweet rice, wheat, white sugar, yellow soybean.

• *Stomach*: barley, bean curd, beef, bitter gourd, black fungus, black pepper, brown sugar, cabbage (Chinese), caraway, carp (gold and grass), celery, chestnut, chicken, chive, clam (saltwater and freshwater), clamshell (river and sea), clove, common button mushroom, corn, crab, cucumber, date (red and black), eggplant, fennel, garlic, ginger (fresh and dried), green onion white head, hawthorn fruit, horse bean, hyacinth bean, kelp, lettuce, licorice, malt, maltose, milk (cow's and human), mung bean, muskmelon, olive, pear, pork, radish, radish leaf, rice bran, rice (polished), salt, shiitake mushroom, squash, sugar cane, sweet basil, sweet rice, sword bean, tangerine, taro, vinegar, water chestnut, watermelon, wheat bran, white pepper, wine.

THE COMMON ACTIONS OF FOODS

The common actions of foods refer to the general actions of foods without referring to any specific internal organ. Many actions are familiar to the Western reader. As an example, the action called "to relieve asthma" means that it is beneficial to asthma patients; the action called "to check perspiration" means that it can reduce perspiration.

Other familiar actions include: to arrest bleeding, to promote blood circulation, to induce bowel movements, to check urination, and so on.

There are also a few actions that are totally unfamiliar to Western readers who do not have backgrounds in Chinese medicine. For instance, what is meant by the terms, "to cool blood" or "to tone up yang"? After reading this book, however, you should have a clear understanding of such actions. Of the large number of actions known in Chinese medicine, less than 100 are commonly used in Chinese diet. Here are actions and effective foods:

• *Arrest bleeding*: black fungus, chestnut, chicken eggshell, cottonseed, cuttlebone, guava, lotus plumule, spinach, vinegar.
• *Calm down the spirits*: licorice, lily flower.
• *Check acid*: chicken eggshell, cuttlebone.
• *Check perspiration*: oyster shell, peach.
• *Check urination*: raspberry.
• *Check seminal ejaculation*: lotus plumule, oyster shell, walnut, black fungus.
• *Counteract toxic effects*: abalone, banana, bean curd, black soybean, castor bean, cherry seed, chicken egg white, Chinese wax gourd, clam (freshwater), cucumber, date (red and black), fig, honey, Job's tears, kohlrabi, radish, salt, sesame oil, small red bean, star fruit, vinegar.
• *Disperse blood coagulations*: brown sugar, chive, chive root, crab, hawthorn fruit, saffron, vinegar.
• *Disperse cold*: ginger (fresh), wine.
• *Eliminate sputum*: Chinese wax gourd, clam (saltwater), longevity fruit, pear, radish, sea grass, seaweed.
• *Facilitate measles eruption*: cherry seed, coriander, sunflower seed.
• *Improve appetite*: green pepper, ham, red pepper.
• *Induce bowel movement*: castor bean, sesame oil.
• *Induce perspiration*: cinnamon twig, coriander, ginger (fresh), green onion leaf, green onion white head, marjoram, rosemary.
• *Lubricate dryness*: bean curd, chicken egg, chicken egg yolk, honey, maltose, milk (human), pear, pork, sesame oil, spinach, sugar cane juice, yellow soybean.
• *Lubricate intestines*: apricot seed (bitter and sweet), banana, milk (cow's), peach, soybean oil, walnut, watermelon.
• *Lubricate lungs*: apple, apricot, chicken egg white, ginseng, lily flower, longevity fruit, loquat, mandarin orange, peanuts, persimmon, strawberry, white fungus, white sugar.
• *Produce fluids*: apple, apricot, bean curd, coconut, date (red and black), ham, lemon, licorice, litchi, maltose, milk (cow's), peach, pear, plum, sour plum, star fruit, strawberry, sugar cane juice, tomato, white fungus, white sugar.
• *Promote blood circulation*: black soybean, brown sugar, chestnut, eel blood, peach, saffron, sweet basil, wine.
• *Promote digestion*: apple, coriander, ginseng, green pepper, hops, malt, nutmeg, papaya, pineapple, plum, radish, radish leaf, red pepper, sweet basil, tomato.
• *Promote energy circulation*: caraway, chive, chive roots, dillseeds, dry mandarin orange peel, fennel, garlic, kumquat, litchi, marjoram, radish leaf, spearmint, star anise, sweet basil, tangerine, tobacco.
• *Promote milk secretion*: common carp, lettuce.
• *Promote urination*: asparagus, barley, Chinese cabbage, carrot, Chinese wax gourd, coconut, coffee, corn, corn silk, cucumber, grape, hops, Job's tears,

kidney bean, lettuce, mandarin orange, mango, mung bean, muskmelon, onion, pineapple, plum, star fruit, sugar cane juice, water chestnut, watermelon.

• *Quench thirst*: crab apple, cucumber, loquat, mango, muskmelon, persimmon, pineapple.

• *Reduce fever*: muskmelon, star fruit, water chestnut.

• *Relieve asthma*: apricot seed (bitter).

• *Relieve cough*: apricot seed (sweet and bitter), kumquat, longevity fruit, mandarin orange, tangerine, thyme.

• *Relieve diarrhea*: guava, sunflower seed.

• *Relieve hot sensations in the body*: chicken egg white, crab, mung bean, sea grass.

• *Relieve pain*: honey, litchi, spearmint, squash, tobacco.

• *Sharpen vision*: abalone, bitter gourd, wild cucumber, freshwater clam, cuttlefish.

• *Soften hardness*: clam (saltwater), kelp, oyster shell, sea grass, seaweed.

• *Tone up blood deficiency*: beef, chicken egg, chicken egg yolk, cuttlefish, milk (human), oyster, spinach.

• *Tone up energy deficiency*: apricot seed (sweet), bean curd, beef, brown sugar, chicken, eel, licorice, maltose, mutton, polished rice, potato, sweet rice, sweet potato.

• *Tone up the heart*: coffee, wheat.

• *Tone up the kidneys*: black sesame seed, string bean, sword bean, wheat, kidneys.

• *Tone up the liver*: black sesame seed, liver.

• *Tone up the lungs*: Job's tears, milk (cow's).

• *Tone up the spleen*: beef, carp (gold), ham, horse bean, hyacinth bean, Job's tears, polished rice, potato, string bean, sweet potato, yellow soybean.

• *Tone up the stomach*: beef, hops, milk (cow's), rosemary.

• *Relieve drunkenness*: apple, ginseng, strawberry.

• *Warm up the internal regions*: black pepper, chicken, chive roots, clove, fennel, ginger (dried), green pepper, mutton, nutmeg, red pepper, sword bean, white pepper.

THE BALANCED DIET IN CHINESE THEORY

Basically, a balanced diet means two different things: First, it means that you should eat foods of various flavors, energies, and organic actions rather than concentrate on a single flavor or energy or organic action. Second, a balanced diet also means that foods are selected according to your needs and physical constitution. The balanced diet in the first sense may be called the *common balanced diet*, and in the second, the *individual's balanced diet*.

It is not easy to eat foods of various energies, flavors, and organic actions, because we are inclined to eat what we like. The foods we like are determined by our taste, which is judged by our mouth and tongue. The mouth and tongue represent only the internal organs of the digestive system. This implies that the foods we like most are pleasing to the organs of the digestive system without considering the internal organs of other body systems (the bladder, liver, kidneys, heart, and others). According to the Chinese theory, sweet foods are pleasing to the stomach and the spleen, pungent foods to the lungs and large intestine, salty foods to the kidneys and bladder, bitter foods to the heart and small intestine, sour foods to the liver and gall bladder.

The foods we enjoy most and eat most frequently are sweet foods, followed by salty foods; therefore, to have a balanced diet, we need to eat more pungent, sour, and bitter foods. This sense of balanced diet is very different from the balanced diet in the Western sense. I have compiled a balanced diet in the Western sense to point out the differences between Chinese and Western balanced diets. The following list of foods represents essential nutrients in Western diet and a comparison from the Chinese point of view.

Western foods: beef for phosphorus; seaweed for iodine; banana for potassium; corn for protein and fat; sweet rice for carbohydrate; celery for calcium; spinach for iron; tomato for vitamin A; potato and chicken liver for vitamin B; lemon for vitamin C; butter for vitamin D; lettuce for vitamin E; honey for vitamin K.

According to Chinese diet, beef is neutral in energy, sweet in flavor, and acts on the spleen and stomach.

Seaweed is cold in energy and salty in flavor, with undetermined organic actions.

Banana is cold in energy and sweet in flavor, with undetermined organic actions.

Corn is neutral in energy and sweet in flavor, and acts on the stomach and large intestine.

Sweet rice is warm in energy and sweet in flavor, and acts on the spleen, the stomach, and lungs.

Celery is neutral in energy and sweet in flavor, and acts on the stomach and liver.

Spinach is cool in energy and sweet in flavor, and acts on the stomach and large intestine.

Tomato is slightly cold in energy and sweet and sour in flavor, with undetermined organic actions.

Potato is neutral in energy and sweet in flavor, with undetermined organic actions. Chicken liver is slightly warm in energy and sweet in flavor, and acts upon the liver and kidneys.

Lemon is extremely sour in flavor, with undetermined energy and organic actions.

Butter is warm in energy and sweet in flavor with undetermined organic actions.

Lettuce is cool in energy and bitter and sweet in flavor, and acts on the stomach and large intestine.

Honey is neutral in energy and sweet in flavor, and acts on the lungs, the spleen, and large intestine.

We can classify all the above foods into groups according to their energies, flavors, and organic actions by ignoring all undetermined items.

• *Cold energy*—seaweed, banana, tomato.
• *Hot energy*—none.
• *Cool energy*—spinach, lettuce.
• *Warm energy*—sweet rice, chicken liver, butter.
• *Neutral energy*—beef, corn, celery, potato, honey.
• *Pungent flavor*—none.
• *Sweet flavor*—beef, banana, corn, sweet rice, celery, spinach, tomato, potato, chicken liver, butter, lettuce, honey.
• *Sour flavor*—tomato, lemon.
• *Salty flavor*—seaweed.
• *Bitter flavor*—lettuce.
• *Acts on the spleen*—beef, sweet rice, honey.
• *Acts on the stomach*—beef, corn, sweet rice, celery, spinach, lettuce.
• *Acts on the large intestine*—corn, spinach, lettuce, honey.
• *Acts on the small intestine*—none.
• *Acts on the liver*—celery, chicken liver.
• *Acts on the gall bladder*—none.
• *Acts on the bladder*—none
• *Acts on the kidneys*—chicken liver.
• *Acts on the heart*—none.
• *Acts on the lungs*—sweet rice, honey.

You can see that in the above, there is no food with a hot energy or with a pungent flavor, and no food to act on the small intestine, gall bladder, bladder, or the heart. Especially, the majority of foods are sweet and act on the spleen, stomach, and large intestine, which are related to the digestive system. Although the foods listed above are selected at random with only Western nutritional balance in mind, they reflect how the Western people eat. Specifically, Westerners eat more sweet foods, which taste good and act predominantly on organs of the digestive system. Small wonder that there are more overweight people in the West than in the East!

THE INDIVIDUAL'S BALANCED DIET

The individual's balanced diet must consider each person's physical constitution. In Chinese diet, there are six different types of physical constitution:

hot, cold, dry, damp, deficient, and excessive. Individuals with different types of physical constitution should follow a different balanced diet. This means that if you have a hot physical constitution, you should eat more cold and cool foods; if you have a cold physical constitution, you should eat more hot and warm foods in order to strike a balance in your body. It is very important, therefore, to know what type of physical constitution you have in order to design a balanced diet for yourself.

A person's physical constitution may be determined in terms of a number of key factors, including subjective sensations, urine, stools, the tongue, and other factors. If you often feel hot, thirsty, and if you normally prefer cold drink and have a reddish complexion, you probably have a *hot* physical constitution. A person with a hot physical constitution may discharge scanty urine (reddish yellow in color) and hard stools. The tongue may appear red with a yellowish coating, but sometimes, the tongue may also appear red with no coating at all.

If you often feel cold and not thirsty, and you normally prefer hot or warm drink and have a pale or whitish complexion, you probably have a *cold* physical constitution. A person with a cold physical constitution may discharge clear urine (that looks white) and soft stools. The tongue of a person with a cold physical constitution normally appears light in color with a thin whitish coating.

If you easily feel thirsty, and your lips, nose, throat, and skin are all dry, and when you cough (when you have a cold) it is mostly dry cough without mucus, then you probably have a *dry* physical constitution. A person with a dry physical constitution may easily have an itch—in the skin or nose or eyes. And he may also display symptoms of constipation, due to the dry conditions of his intestines. A person with a dry physical constitution is normally skinny and cannot gain weight easily.

If you feel heavy in the body and very often tired and if your tongue appears glossy and greasy, then you probably have a *damp* physical constitution. A person with a damp physical constitution easily becomes overweight due to water retention, called edema. This type of person may look fat but is rather weak in energy. The Chinese believe that to remove water from the body, it is necessary for this type of person to promote urination and induce perspiration and to eat aromatic foods, which are believed to have the effects of drying the internal region.

Another type of physical constitution is called *deficient*. A person with a deficient physical constitution is weak in energy and normally in low spirits. This type of person may have a pale complexion, feel tired very often, perspire excessively, have palpitations or shortness of breath. The tongue may appear clean and light without a coating. A person with a deficient physical constitution is underweight or skinny, and often suffers from falling symptoms (falling of the stomach, prolapse of the uterus, prolapse of the anus), which are caused by energy deficiency. The body does not have sufficient energy to support the internal organs, so the organs begin to fall.

The last type of physical constitution is called *excessive*. A person with an excessive physical constitution is strong and energetic and often in high spirits, and speaks in a high-pitched voice. This type of person normally has a reddish complexion and may suffer from constipation, hypertension, or heart disease. Because the body has accumulated too much energy, traffic jams are created leading to blockages of various kinds. It must be emphasized here, however, people usually have a mixed physical constitution—cold and dry, damp and hot, cold and deficient, or another combination.

The individual's balanced diet, therefore, is always a mixture of foods with different flavors and energies suited to the needs of the individual's physical constitution. To design a balanced diet for yourself, there are some general principles you can follow: If you have a cold physical constitution, eat more foods with a hot or warm energy and fewer foods with a cold or cool energy. As for the flavors of foods, eat more sweet and pungent foods and decrease bitter foods.

If you have a hot physical constitution, eat more foods with a cool or cold energy; considering food flavors, eat more bitter foods and fewer pungent ones. If you have a dry physical constitution, eat more foods that lubricate dryness (honey, for example) and avoid foods that dry dampness in the body (such as small red beans).

If you have a damp physical constitution, eat more foods that dry dampness and promote water passage; avoid foods that can produce fluids. If you have a deficient physical constitution, you should eat more foods that can move you towards the excessive side in energy. Such foods are called tonics (yam and red date, for example); eat fewer foods that can make you deficient (these normally taste bitter). If you have an excessive physical constitution, choose more foods that can promote energy and blood circulation; avoid foods that can increase your energy.

I have discussed how the individual's balanced diet may be designed according to six types of individual physical constitution. In addition, each person should also pay attention to a diet that maintains the balance of internal organs. This is called the organic balanced diet.

THE ORGANIC BALANCED DIET

The organic balanced diet refers to a diet that maintains the balance of internal organs. Since each person has different organic conditions, the organic balanced diet also varies with these conditions. Each individual has organic strengths and organic weaknesses. For example, a person may be strong in the digestive functions but weak in the reproductive functions. The fact that a person has an excellent appetite does not necessarily mean that his heart is also in good shape or his sexual capacities measure up to the standard.

Ideally, the diet for organic balance guarantees that all internal organs are kept in good condition. This is important, not only because all internal organs should be in good shape, but also because when one organ is excessively strong, it tends to weaken another organ, creating an organic imbalance. Here is a simple example: When a person gains twenty or thirty pounds within two or three months, he may become sexually weak or even impotent. Why? Because the excessive strength of his stomach is putting pressure on his kidneys, which, according to Chinese medical theory, are responsible for sexual capacities.

It is rather difficult for a layman to determine personal organic strengths and weaknesses that require expert knowledge about Chinese medicine. Suppose as an example, a person suffering from heartburn consults his doctor and is advised to have a physical checkup that may turn up nothing—no gastritis, gastric ulcers, or excessive gastric acid. His stomach may also look normal, so the doctor tells him that he is in good health. But then the person suffering with heartburn begins to wonder whether he really is in good health. A question emerges in his mind, "If I am in good health, why do I have heartburn?"

Let's assume this person is quite curious and one day decides to consult a Chinese herbalist. The Chinese herbalist asks him how his stomach feels and he answers that he feels burning sensations in his stomach. The Chinese herbalist asks him whether he enjoys drinking liquor, and he replies that drinking whiskey produces even more severe hot sensations in his stomach. The Chinese herbalist asks him whether spicy foods agree with him, and he answers that spicy foods make his hot sensations worse. The Chinese herbalist then diagnoses that the patient's stomach is too hot. But the patient insists that his doctor checked his stomach very thoroughly and found nothing wrong with his stomach.

How does the Chinese herbalist know that this person's stomach is too hot? In fact, the answer is not as difficult as it appears. The fact that the patient feels burning sensations in the stomach indicates that this is a hot disease which gets worse when consuming liquor and spicy foods. Both liquor and spicy foods are either very warm or hot—bad for a hot stomach. A hot stomach should be cooled down by eating foods that have a cold or cool energy. If such foods cannot heal the symptoms, then cold herbs should be used; herbs are stronger than foods. This brings out another important aspect of balanced diet, namely, the diet for restoring the balance of the body.

RESTORING THE BODY BALANCE

When a person becomes ill, the balance of his or her body is lost—at least temporarily. If you have a headache, for example, it means your body balance is lost; it is necessary to create a diet to restore the balance, or in other words, to relieve your symptoms. Normally, the symptoms you develop are consistent with your physical constitution: If you have a hot physical constitution, you will probably develop hot symptoms (such as skin eruptions and hot rheumatism), a cold physical constitution, cold symptoms (such as cold vomiting and cold rheumatism). For this reason, it is important to know your own physical constitution to deal with occasional symptoms. Conversely, it is also easy for you to identify your physical constitution through the symptoms. If you have a tendency to suffer from constipation, you most probably have a hot or dry physical constitution; if you suffer from rheumatic pain that gets worse on cold days or on exposure to cold environments, then you most probably have a cold physical constitution. People who suffer rheumatic pain in the same joints—with increasing pain on rainy days—have damp rheumatism. These people probably have a damp physical constitution.

The symptoms may sometimes run counter to one's physical constitution, however, which means that a person with a hot physical constitution may develop cold symptoms from time to time, and a person with a cold physical constitution may develop hot symptoms as well. As an example, even though you have a hot physical constitution, you may still suffer from cold vomiting (a cold symptom); and even though you have a cold physical constitution, sometimes you may still have fever (a hot symptom). For this reason, treatment of symptoms may involve foods that are normally not good for the person who develops the temporary symptoms. When a person with a cold physical constitution develops fever (a hot symptom), he or she may have to eat foods with a cold energy, although such foods may normally be bad for that person.

The more you learn about Chinese diet, the more you will be able to apply it with flexibility. Even with a fair knowledge of the Chinese beliefs, you will benefit from it. How would you feel if you recovered from eczema simply by drinking mung bean soup for a few weeks? How would you feel if you recovered from neuralgic pain simply by drinking hot ginger soup? How would you feel if you recovered from migraine headache simply by drinking peppermint tea?

I had runny nose yesterday and my eyes were itchy. I knew I had caught cold—but I did not have cold sensations nor did I have fever. The only symptoms were runny nose and itchy eyes. So, I boiled hot water, cut up a lemon, squeezed juice into the hot water and added one spoonful of sugar. I drank the warm lemon juice. At this writing I feel fine. Why did I drink lemon juice? Everybody knows that lemon has lots of vitamin C. But yesterday, I was not interested in vitamin C, I only wanted to stop my nasal discharge. I know that lemon is extremely sour and the foods that have a sour flavor are obstructive. This is why I used lemon juice—its obstructive nature can stop my runny nose. Moreover, lemon can produce fluids that are good for me, not only because my eyes were itchy (due to dryness) but also because

I have a dry physical constitution. Why did I add sugar? There are two reasons: One, lemon juice is so sour that it is not very pleasing to me; two, sugar can also produce fluids that are good for my dry symptom. I could have made a mistake by adding honey instead of sugar; honey is very glossy, which could make my nasal discharge worse and cancel out the obstructive nature of lemon. Why did I drink very warm lemon juice instead of chilling it in the refrigerator and drinking it cold? Because my runny nose was caused by coldness and I knew the warm lemon juice would make me warm.

3

Body Types and the Yin-Yang Principles

In the previous chapters, I discussed energies and flavors of foods. Now you can put this knowledge to use. But before you begin to apply my suggestions to benefit your health, there is one important concept you should know about—yin and yang. The theory of yin and yang is fundamental in Chinese medicine and should be regarded as such when discussing food cures. In fact, everything in the universe can be classified into yin and yang: man is yang, woman is yin; the sun is yang, the moon is yin; day is yang, night is yin; functions of the human body are yang, its shape is yin; heaven is yang, earth is yin; skin and muscles are yang, internal organs are yin; the back is yang, the abdomen is yin.

The energies and flavors of foods are also classified into yin and yang. Hot and warm energies are yang; cool and cold energies are yin. Pungent and sweet flavors are yang; sour, bitter, and salty flavors are yin. When we try to classify foods into yin and yang, we must consider both their energies and flavors. Sometimes, the energy of a food may be yang and its flavor yin, which seems contradictory but is not.

Y-SCORES

I have designed a comprehensive chart of y-scores (Table 1) by which foods and body types, diseases, moods, and four seasons may be classified into yin and yang. Y-scores stand for the yin or yang scores of a given item. This table is not only simple in design but also accurate to apply. After you have learned how to use the table by reading this chapter, you will find it very convenient to use in deciding what foods to eat and under what circumstances to eat them.

Y-scores can be used to determine to what extent a given food or disease or body type or season is yin or yang because it is a quantification of yin and yang. If a given item is preceded by $+$, it is yang; if preceded by $-$, it is yin.

TABLE 1 COMPREHENSIVE Y-SCORES

			YANG		YIN	
	Energies of foods	hot	warm	neutral	cool	cold
	Y-scores	+8	+4	0	−4	−8
	Flavors of foods	pungent	sweet	light	sour salty	bitter
	Y-scores	+8	+4	0	−4 −6	−8
	Movements of foods	outward	upwards	neutral	downwards	inward
	Y-scores	+8	+4	0	−4	−8
Individual Body Types	**Hot-cold**	hot	warm	neutral	cool	cold
	Y-scores	+8	+4	0	−4	−8
	Dry-damp	dry (underweight)		neutral	damp (overweight)	
	Y-scores	+8 +7 +5 +4 +3 +2 +1		0	−1 −2 −3 −4 −5 −6 −7 −8	
	Excessive-deficient	normally energetic	normally not tired	neutral	normally lazy	normally tired
	Y-scores	+8	+4	0	−4	−8
	Dispositions	restless or impatient	fairly active	neutral	fairly relaxed	easy-going or patient
	Y-scores	+8	+4	0	−4	−8
	Sex life	very high sex drive	sex > foods	neutral	foods > sex	very low sex drive
	Y-scores	+8	+4	0	−4	−8
	Moods	cheerful or joyful	hopeful or comfortable	thinking or reasoning	depressed or sad	scary or fearful
	Y-scores	+8	+4	0	−4	−8
	Four seasons	summer	spring	summer-autumn	autumn	winter
	Y-scores	+8	+4	0	−4	−8

Yin and yang may be better understood as two adjectives, instead of nouns, because as adjectives, we can say one thing is more yang or more yin than another. For example, if the energy of a food is hot, it has a y-score of +8, and if the energy of another food is warm, it has a y-score of +4, which means that the first food is more yang than the second one. Again, if the energy of one food is cool, it has a y-score of −4, and if the energy of another food is cold, it has a y-score of −8, which means the second food is more yin than the first one.

In determining the y-score of a given food, both the y-score of its energy and that of its flavor should be taken into account. To compute it, the y-scores of flavor and those of energy of a given food should be calculated separately; then add them and divide by 2 to arrive at the y-score. As an example, garlic has a warm energy and a pungent flavor. It has a y-score of $+4$ in energy and $+8$ in flavor with a total score of $+12$ ($4 + 8$), which means garlic has a y-score of $+6$. Take watermelon as another example; it has a cold energy and a sweet flavor. This means that watermelon has a y-score of -8 in energy and $+4$ in flavor with the total score of -4, which means watermelon has a y-score of -2.

If a given food has two or more flavors or energies, their y-scores should average out to the mean score. As an example, kumquat has three flavors, namely, pungent ($+8$), sweet ($+4$), and sour (-4), with a total score of $+8$, which averages out to $+3$ as its flavor; and since kumquat is warm ($+4$), you add it to $+3$ (flavor average) and divide by 2. The y-score of kumquat is $+3$ or $+4$.

TABLE 2   Y-SCORES OF FOODS

	YANG			YIN	
Energy of foods	hot	warm	neutral	cool	cold
Y-scores	+8	+4	0	−4	−8
Flavor of foods	pungent	sweet	light	sour salty	bitter
Y-scores	+8	+4	0	−4 −6	−8

After determining the y-score of a given food, you can know its movements simply by reading Table 3.

TABLE 3   Y-SCORES OF MOVEMENTS OF FOODS

	YANG			YIN	
Movements of foods	outward	upwards	neutral	downwards	inward
Y-scores	+8	+4	0	−4	−8

If a food has a y-score of $+8$, it can move outward; if it has a y-score of $+4$, it can move upwards; if it has a y-score of -4, it can move downwards; if it has a y-score of -8, it can move inward; if it has a y-score of 0, it is neutral. What if a food has a y-score of $+6$? Does it move upwards or outward? To answer this question, it is important to remember that there is a continuity between yin and yang which, in turn, means there is also a continuity between upward and outward movements. If a food has a y-score of $+6$, it may move upwards and outward simultaneously, or it may move more upwards than outward or vice versa. As we have just seen, garlic has a y-score of $+6$ and watermelon has a y-score of -2. With this information, we know that garlic moves upwards or outward but that watermelon moves downwards. This is the general principle governing the relationships between energy and flavor of foods on the one hand and the movements of foods on the other. There are exceptions to this general principle, which are usually stated in this book under each food involved. One such exception is sword bean. According to the general principle, sword bean should move upwards since it is warm and sweet. Nevertheless, sword bean moves downwards instead of upwards according to the established theory.

As already discussed in the previous chapter, many health problems are classified into outward, upward, downward, inward diseases, symptoms, or ailments. Vomiting, panting, and hiccupping are upward ailments; prolapse of anus and falling of the stomach are downward problems; fever, excessive perspiration, and night sweat are outward symptoms; diarrhea and abdominal swelling are inward ailments. Certainly exceptions exist, but as a general rule, foods that have a y-score of $+4$ (upward movement) may be used to treat downward diseases; foods that have a y-score of -4 (downward movement) may be used to treat upward diseases; foods that have a y-score of $+8$ (outward movement) may be used to treat inward diseases; and foods that have a y-score of -8 (inward movement) may be used to treat outward diseases.

Suppose you are hiccupping at this moment and try to decide whether to eat garlic or watermelon to stop the hiccupping. It is obvious that watermelon should be your logical choice: It has a y-score of -2, which means that it can move downwards; that is good for hiccupping. Let's further assume that you have a mild cold and try to decide whether to eat garlic or watermelon in order to speed up your recovery. It is obvious that garlic should be your logical choice, because it has a y-score of $+6$, which means that it can move upwards and outward to induce perspiration; thus it is good for a common cold.

The movements of foods may also be applied to treat the diseases that are not in motion, namely, they are not moving upwards or downwards or outward or inward, but stay in the same region. For example, if you have a headache, the pain may stay in your head without moving in any direction; if you have a stomachache, the pain may stay in the stomach without moving in any direction; if you suffer from arthritis, the pain may stay in the knee joint without moving in any direction. Such symptoms are called symptoms in the fixed regions, and they may be treated by foods with different y-scores: When a disease occurs in the upper region, like headache or stomachache, it should be treated by foods with a y-score of $+4$ (upward movement) so that the effects of foods can reach the head; when a disease occurs in the lower region, like arthritis involving the knee joints, it should be treated by foods with a y-score of -4 (downward movement) so that the foods can reach the knee joints; when a disease occurs in the outer region, like pain in the muscles, it should be treated by foods with a y-score of +8 (outward movement) so that the foods can reach the muscles; when a disease occurs in the inner region, like constipation or abdominal swelling, it should be treated by foods with a y-score of −8 (inward movement) so that the foods can reach the affected regions.

YOUR BODY TYPE

What if you are not suffering from any disease? What foods should you eat? To choose foods wisely, it is necessary to have an adequate knowledge of your body type. Body types, like foods, may also be classified into yin and yang to be determined by the concept of y-scores. If your body type has a y-score of, say, +8, it is wise for you to eat more foods with a y-score of −8 to strike a balance; if you have a y-score of −8, for example, it is wise to eat more foods with a y-score of +8 to strike a balance. In other words, a yin person wisely should eat more yang foods and a yang person more yin foods to create a balance between yin and yang in the body.

But how can you determine your body type, whether it is yin or yang? There are four basic factors that should be taken into consideration: hot/cold, dry/damp, dispositions, and sex life.

TABLE 4   YIN AND YANG BODY TYPES

Body Types	YANG			YIN	
Hot-cold	hot	warm	neutral	cool	cold
Y-scores	+8	+4	0	−4	−8
Dry-damp	dry (underweight)		neutral	damp (overweight)	
Y-scores	+8 +7 +6 +5 +4 +3 +2 +1		0 −1 −2	−3 −4 −5 −6 −7 −8	
Excessive-deficient	normally energetic	normally not tired	neutral	normally lazy	normally tired
Y-scores	+8	+4	0	−4	−8
Disposi-tions	restless or impatient	fairly active	neutral	fairly relaxed	easy-going or patient
Y-scores	+8	+4	0	−4	−8
Sex life	very high sex drive	sex>foods	neutral	foods>sex	very low sex drive
Y-scores	+8	+4	0	−4	−8

The hot/cold dichotomy may be determined by the answers to the following four questions:

First, do you normally have cold hands or cold feet? If your answer is yes, then your y-score is −8.

Second, do you normally have warm hands or warm feet? If your answer is yes, then your y-score is +8.

Third, do you generally prefer cold winter to hot summer? If your answer is yes, then your y-score is −4.

Fourth, do you generally prefer hot summer to cold winter? If your answer is yes, then your y-score is +4.

If you cannot decide on the answer to any of the above questions, then your y-score is 0 (neutral). Let's assume that your answers to the first and third questions are positive, then your y-score, the addition of −8 and −4 divided by 2, is −6.

The dry/damp dichotomy may be determined by your body weight, with each 5 overweight or underweight pounds to be counted as +1 or −1, making a maximum score of either +8 or −8. Here's how it works: If you are 5 pounds overweight, your y-score is −1; if you are 5 pounds underweight, your y-score is +1; if you are 10 pounds overweight, your y-score is −2; if you are 40 pounds (or more) overweight, your y-score is −8. As you can see, overweight is yin, underweight is yang. Men are yang and women are yin (small wonder there are more overweight women than men); a rooster is a very yang creature (small wonder that each rooster is underweight); a hen is a very yin creature (small wonder that each hen is overweight). One man may be more underweight than another, because the former is more yang than the latter; by the same token, a woman may be more overweight than another, because the former is more yin than the latter.

The dichotomy of excess and deficiency may be determined by the conditions of body energy. If you normally feel energetic, your y-score is +8; if you seldom feel tired, but only once in a while, your y-score is +4; if you normally feel lazy but not tired, your y-score is −4; if you normally feel tired, your y-score is −8; if you do not know the answer, your y-score is 0. If both +8 and +4 are applicable to you, pick +8 as your y-score; if both −8 and −4 are applicable to you, pick −8 as your y-score; if more than two scores are applicable to you, average them out to arrive at a y-score.

The dichotomy of dispositions may be determined by the nature of your answer to this question: Do you fall to sleep while you are on board a plane or sitting in a chair or in the car as a passenger? If your answer is "very often or easily," your y-score is −8; if your answer is "never or only when extremely tired," your y-score is +8; if your answer is "easily when a little tired," your y-score is +4; if your answer is "occasionally even though not tired," your y-score is −4. If both +4 and +8 are applicable to you, pick +8; if both −4 and −8 are applicable to you, pick −8.

The dichotomy of sex life is self-evident, requiring no further explanations with the exception of the greater than symbol (>), which is used here to denote preference. Sex > foods denotes enjoyment of sex more than foods, which has a y-score of +4; and foods > sex denotes enjoyment of foods more than sex, which has a y-score of −4. In case two scores are equally applicable to you, pick the higher score as your y-score. As an example, if both +4 and +8 are applicable to you, your y-score should be +8; if both -4 and -8 are applicable to you, your y-score should be -8. If you cannot decide on which category you belong to, your y-score is 0, which means neutral or indecisive.

After you have arrived at a y-score in each of the above five dichotomies, add the five y-scores and then divide by 5 to arrive at your y-score—a description of *your body type*. For example, if your y-score in the hot/cold dichotomy +4, in the dry/damp dichotomy +8, in the excessive/deficient dichotomy +8, in the dispositions dichotomy 0, and in the sex life dichotomy +4, then your y-scores should average out to +5. This is the y-score of your body type.

You are ready to choose foods for your needs on this basic principle: A person with a yang body type should eat more yin foods and a person with a yin body type should eat more yang foods in order to create a yin-yang balance in the body.

ALLERGIES AND BODY TYPES

All of us have heard about the word "allergy" in modern medicine, but what does it mean? Some people cannot stand certain foods, and they are often told by their doctors that they cannot stand such foods because they are allergic to them. Thus the word allergy, in fact, is nothing but a vicious circle in disguise, neither better nor worse than no explanation at all.

The concept of allergies in modern medicine may be explained better in terms of the interaction between foods and body types, however. An individual with a body type y-score of −8 for example, may not tolerate foods with a y-score of −8, because they will drive him towards the yin limit; an individual with a y-score of +8 in body type may not tolerate foods with a y-score of +8, because they will drive him towards the yang limit, particularly when such foods are consumed for a prolonged period of time. If your body type has a y-score of +8, it is better for you to eat more seaweed, for example, which has a y-score of −6 than fresh ginger, which has a y-score of +6; fresh ginger adds +6 to your body and makes a total y-score of +14; by eating seaweed, −6 is added to your body, which makes only a total of +2. Thus, the choice of eating seaweed and fresh ginger equals the difference between +14 and +2, indeed, a very significant difference. It is important, therefore, to select foods according to your body type so that a balance between yin and yang may be created in the body to maintain good health and to prevent disease.

DISEASES AND Y-SCORES

The hot/cold dichotomy concept may be applied to disease as well, because some diseases are hot, while others are cold diseases. Here are the criteria to help you distinguish between the two: If the disease gets worse on exposure to cold surroundings or if it gets better on exposure to warm or hot surrounding, then it is a cold disease and should be assigned a y-score of −8; if the disease deteriorates on exposure to warm or hot surroundings or if it gets better on exposure to cool or cold surroundings, then it is a hot disease and should be assigned a y-score of +8. If the patient prefers cool or cold surroundings, it is a warm disease, which should be assigned a y-score of +4; if the patient prefers warm or hot surroundings, it is a cool disease and should be assigned a y-score of −4. In case both +4 and +8 are applicable to a patient, +8 should be chosen as its y-score; in case both −4 and −8 are applicable to a patient, −8 should be chosen as its y-score. In case a patient cannot decide on the right answer, the y-score is 0.

The y-scores of diseases may be applied to choose foods for patients the same way the y-scores of body types are applied to choose foods for different people. When a person has a high fever (obviously a hot disease), it is only logical for him to eat more yin foods; conversely, if a person is shivering with cold, it is only logical for him to eat more yang foods. Some arthritis patients get worse in winter, which means that it is a cold disease; therefore, they should eat more yang foods. If some people have a skin disease that gets worse in summer, on exposure to sunlight or heat in the kitchen, it is a hot disease; they should eat more yin foods to improve the conditions. In my clinical practice, I have seen patients with skin itch (like urticaria) which starts as soon as they come close to the kitchen as if they were allergic to the kitchen. In fact, they are not allergic to the kitchen; it is the kitchen heat that triggers their itch. Conversely, some patients with itchy skin feel much better when they are in the kitchen; but as soon as they are exposed to cold air, their itching starts, because they are suffering from a cold disease.

MOODS AND Y-SCORES

Moreover, our knowledge of food y-scores also enables us to control our moods—or create moods we desire. As you can see from the chart, cheerful and joyful moods have a y-score of +8, hopeful and comfortable a y-score of +4, thinking and reasoning a y-score of 0, depressed and sad moods have a y-score of −4, scary and fearful moods a y-score of −8. Assume that you feel depressed and sad, for one reason or another, and begin to wonder, "Which food will change my depressed or sad moods—garlic or watermelon?" The answer seems clear from the chart: Garlic should be your logical choice, because it can increase your yang scores and shift your moods towards the yang side.

There is another example demonstrating how to create the moods by eating suitable foods. People often say, "I can't think straight." To think straight, the y-score of moods should be 0, as indicated in the chart; foods with a neutral energy and light flavor are the most suitable foods to eat.

TABLE 5   Y-SCORES OF MOODS

Moods	YANG			YIN	
	cheerful/ joyful	hopeful/ comfortable	thinking/ reasoning	depressed/ sad	scary/ fearful
Y-scores	+8	+4	0	−4	−8

It is important to remember, however, that the above examples are given merely from the point of view of y-scores of foods. In actual practice, we must also consider y-scores of our body types. For example, if your body type has a y-score of +8 and you eat the foods with a y-score of +8, your body conditions will stay in the same position, namely, a y-score of +8 that creates cheerful and joyful moods instead of thinking and reasoning ones. On the other hand, if you eat the foods with a y-score of −8, it will shift your body conditions from +8 towards 0 to create thinking and reasoning moods.

The formula that creates the desired moods may be stated as follows: Y-score of moods equals the addition of y-score of body type and y-score of foods divided by 2. By using this formula, a person with a body type y-score of +4 should eat foods with a y-score of +4 to create hopeful and comfortable moods; a person with body type y-score of −4 should eat foods with a y-score of +4 to create the moods conducive to thinking and reasoning.

According to the y-scores of Table 5, it seems impossible for a person with a body type y-score of −8 to have cheerful and joyful moods no matter which foods he or she eats. This conclusion is wrong. "Body type" refers only to a relatively constant state of physical conditions that may change occasionally to create a different mood. When we say, "He is a cheerful person," we are talking about the constant mood consistent with his body type; but when we say, "He is cheerful," we mean the temporary mood (that may not be consistent with his body type) created by a combination of body type and foods or a temporary change in body conditions due to other environmental factors.

Y-SCORES AND THE FOUR SEASONS

Is it true that a person with a body type y-score of +4, for example, always or frequently remains hopeful and comfortable and that a person with a y-score of −4 is always or frequently in a depressed or sad mood? The answer depends mostly on what he eats as well as on other environmental factors. We have to eat and live in some environment. Our body begins to interact with the foods and surroundings, which combine to create different moods.

The four seasons are environmental factors that can significantly affect our moods. Like foods, the four seasons are also classified into yin and yang with different y-scores assigned to them: summer, +8; spring, +4; autumn, −4; winter, −8.

TABLE 6   Y-SCORES OF FOUR SEASONS

	YANG			YIN	
Seasons	summer	spring	summer-autumn	autumn	winter
Y-scores	+8	+4	0	−4	−8

In summer, people of all body types move towards the yang side, in winter, towards the yin side, hence creating seasonal moods. So in summer it is easier to create cheerful and joyful moods, and in winter to become depressed and sad or even scared and fearful.

It is important to remember, whichever your body type, you should eat more hot and pungent foods in summer, more warm and sweet foods in spring, more neutral and light foods in between summer and autumn, more cool and sour foods in autumn, and more cold and bitter foods in winter. This may seem to contradict the principle stated earlier that to create the yin-yang balance people with a hot body type should eat more cold foods and people with a cold body type more hot foods, which implies that one should eat more cold foods in summer, more hot in winter to create a yin-yang balance. Nevertheless, the two seemingly contradictory principles are resolved by the fact that foods and seasons have a difference in their impact on the human body: Foods, when eaten, become part of the human body; the four seasons (as environmental factors) are external to the human body. When a person with a hot body type eats cold foods, for example, the cold energy of foods is absorbed to become part of his body so that the heat of the body is reduced and the yin-yang balance within the body is achieved; on the other hand, summer heat is always external to the body and in summer, the body surface is constantly under the impact of summer heat that creates an imbalance between the internal body region and the body surface; for this reason, in summer, it is necessary to eat more hot and warm foods to increase internal body heat so that a yin-yang balance between the internal region and body surface can be achieved. By the same token, in winter, the body surface is constantly under the impact of winter cold that creates an imbalance between the internal region and the body surface, and it is necessary to eat more cold and cool foods to cool the internal region to achieve a yin-yang balance between the internal body region and the surface.

Chinese herbalists believe that in spring, one should eat more foods that move upwards (warm and sweet foods) to stay in harmony with the growing season (living things begin to grow, an upward movement); in summer, eat more foods that move outward (hot and pungent foods) to remain harmonious with the season (living things begin to expand, an outward movement); in autumn, eat more foods that move downwards (cool and sour foods) (living things begin to fall, a downward movement); in winter, eat more foods that move inward (cold, salty, and bitter foods) (living things begin to shrink, an inward movement). This theory is consistent with the common practice of applying fertilizers to plants in spring when living things begin to grow, but futile to do in winter when plants are ready to move downwards.

I take this principle of harmony between foods and the four seasons very seriously, not only because I practice Chinese medicine, but also because of a painful personal experience. I used to develop swelling and pain in my foot every winter. Each recurrence brought severe pain, and the swelling lasted for a month or longer, virtually preventing me from walking and working. At first, I kept asking myself why this happened only in winter, not in summer. I figured that it must have something to do with the winter cold. So I started warming my foot in hot water every day, which seemed to help a little bit but not enough to cure the pain or heal the swelling to any significant degree. This problem lasted for three years. One day, this principle of harmony between the internal region and body surface suddenly dawned on me. I began to suspect the swelling and pain could have developed from the disparity between my internal region and body surface since the body surface was constantly exposed to severe winter cold whereas my internal region remained hot. When a disparity between the internal region and body surface developed, the heat in the internal region erupted like a volcano, the cause of the pain and swelling. When I tried to warm my foot in hot water, I tried to counteract the cold impact of winter on my body surface instead of staying in harmony with the winter by cooling down my internal region. So I began to eat yin foods and yin herbs and finally bade farewell to those annual miseries, thanks to the master Chinese herbalist Shi-Chen Li (1518–1593). He stated, in his most celebrated book in Chinese herbal therapy, *An Outline of Materia Medica*, published in 1578: "In spring, one should eat more pungent and warm foods to stay in harmony with the upward movement of the season; in summer, one should eat more pungent and hot foods to stay in harmony with the outward movement of the season; in autumn, one should eat more sour and warm foods to stay in harmony with the downward movement of the season; in winter, one should eat more bitter and cold foods to stay in harmony with the inward movement of the season."

4
Spices and Herbs

In this and the five following chapters, each food includes Indications (under the heading), Description, Applications, Clinical reports, Experiments (when there are any), and Remarks. The information is understandable, except for the Description, which includes energy, flavor, actions of foods and vital internal organs affected. If, for example, the words "spleen and stomach" are listed, it means that this food will affect the spleen and the stomach. When a food has more than one flavor, they are listed as "sweet and sour" or "pungent and sweet," or another combination. The food actions are usually stated as "warming up the stomach," "cooling down the blood," and other terms. The dosages prescribed under Applications are approximate. You should apply them with flexibility, depending on your body size and height. If you are heavier or taller, for example, the dosages may be increased accordingly, and vice versa. If in doubt, or in case of more serious symptoms, it is always wise and necessary to consult your own physician.

Star Anise

Hernia, abdominal pain, lumbago, beriberi, vomiting.

Description: warm; pungent and sweet; warms up yang energy (energy that travels in the skin and muscles as opposed to yin energy that travels through internal organs) and promotes energy circulation; affects the spleen, kidneys, and liver.

Applications: Crush 7 star anises and 7 fresh onion white heads, and boil them in 3 cups water over low heat until liquid is reduced to 1 cup. Drink it like tea, twice a day, to cure constipation, urination difficulty, and abdominal swelling.

• Bake 40 g star anise and grind into powder; drink 5 g of the powder dissolved in warm rice wine each time, twice a day, to relieve hernia of the small intestine.

• Fry star anise and grind into powder; dissolve 7 g of the powder with a little salt in warm water before meals, twice a day, to cure lumbago.

Remarks: According to traditional Chinese theory, star anise heals all sorts of cold symptoms, as well as hernia, swollen scrotum, lumbago, and beriberi. It is wise to take star anise with a little salt, rice wine, and cinnamon for better results. If you have an eye or skin disease, you should avoid star anise.

Fennel Seed

Hernia, cold pain in lower abdomen, lumbago, stomachache, vomiting, dry and wet beriberi.

Description: warm; pungent; warms the internal region and promotes energy circulation; affects the kidneys, the bladder, and stomach.

Applications: Prepare 40 g apricot seeds; crush 20 g fresh green onion white heads with roots and bake until dry; prepare 40 g fennel seed; grind all the ingredients into a powder. Drink 10 g of the powder dissolved in rice wine each time, twice a day, to relieve pain in hernia of small intestine.

• Fry equal amounts of fennel and litchi seeds and grind into powder; dissolve 10 g of the powder in rice wine and drink each time, twice a day, to relieve pain in hernia of the small intestine.

• Measure equal amounts fennel and black pepper and grind them into powder; dissolve 10 g of the powder in rice wine each time, twice a day, to relieve pain in small intestine.

• For lumbago, when unable to turn sideways, and extreme fatigue, cook slices of pork kidneys with fried fennel and eat at meals.

• To heal cold stomachache and abdominal pain, use fennel and ginger as seasonings when preparing meals.

Clinical reports: For treatment of incarcerated hernia of small intestine, use 10 to 20 g fennel (less for children) to make tea; drink it hot; if no effects are shown within 15 to 30 minutes, repeat once more. Or, use hot water to make fennel soup (4 to 8 g fennel seed for adults and 2 g for children), and drink the soup; 10 minutes later, repeat and drink once more, then lie down on your back with your legs together and knees half bent for 40 minutes. In general, the incarcerated hernia should restore itself within half an hour, and the pain should disappear or improve, otherwise, surgery is indicated, according to this clinical report. Among the 26 cases treated from 2 hours to 3 days, 22 cases have recovered and 4 cases have shown no effects (3 cases of incarcerated omentum majus and 1 case of parietal necrosis). The report also indicates that the treatment results are better in cases with a shorter history of the disease; if the symptoms have a long history, necrosis and perforation may have already occurred and they should not be treated by this method.

In case of incarcerated omentum majus, surgery should be considered, according to this report.

• For treatment of hydrocele of tunica vaginalis and elephantiasis scroti: Fry 16 g fennel and 5 g salt until black; grind them into powder to make cakes with 2 raw duck eggs; eat the cakes while drinking warm rice wine at bedtime. Each treatment program continues for 4 days; the second treatment program begins 2 to 5 days after completing the first program. Treatment may continue, if necessary. Among the 64 cases of hydrocele of tunica vaginalis treated for 1 to 6 programs, 59 cases recovered, 1 case has shown progress, 4 cases have shown no results. The majority of patients suffering from elephantiasis scroti have shown results only after 4 treatment programs; the results are rather satisfactory with no side effects (except the cases in which the scrotum was as hard as stone).

Remarks: Chinese herbalists believe that fennel travels very fast in the body and it can quickly warm up the internal region. Therefore, fennel can treat cold pain in the body; but since it is warm in nature, fennel should not be used to treat any hot disease, such as hot diarrhea or pain that occurs on exposure to hot surroundings (sunburn, burn, or warm temperatures). Fennel is not recommended for men with excessively strong erection and premature ejaculation. Fennel should be of the best quality, fresh and aromatic; it is considered an aromatic digestive and carminative, good for regulation of intestines, expelling intestinal gas, warming up internal region, and exciting the nervous system. Fennel root is warm, and tastes pungent and sweet, it can warm the kidneys and promote energy circulation to relieve pain; good for cold pain in hernia, cold vomiting, abdominal pain, and arthritis.

Sweet Basil

Headache in common cold, diarrhea, indigestion, stomachache, irregular menstruation.

Description: warm; pungent; promotes energy, blood circulation, and digestion; affects the lungs, spleen, stomach, and large intestine.

Applications: Use sweet basil leaves as a seasoning to substitute for parsley or green onion for relief of headache in common cold.

• There are 2 ways sweet basil may be used to relieve menstrual pain: Cook a few leaves with chicken egg and consume it as a soup with some rice wine (good for women with premenstrual pain); another way is to cook a few sweet basil leaves with ginger, green onion, and some meats or fish (good for menstrual pain due to coldness).

• Sweet basil, fresh ginger, and licorice may be boiled in water; drink it like tea to cure acute gastroenteritis, abdominal swelling, and pain.

Dillseed

Abdominal pain, poor appetite, shortage of milk secretion after childbirth.

Description: warm; pungent; warms the body, promotes energy circulation, and counteracts fish and meat poisoning; affects the spleen and kidneys.

Applications: Fry dillseeds until aromatic and grind into powder; dissolve 5 g of the powder in warm rice wine and drink each time to cure lumbago due to twisted muscles.

Remarks: Dill leaf is warm, pungent, and oppressive. According to 1 experiment, dill leaf is found to have the effect of lowering blood pressure and expanding blood vessels in animals.

Cinnamon Bark

Cold limbs, abdominal pain, diarrhea, hot sensations in the upper region with cold sensations in the lower region.

Description: hot; pungent and sweet; affects the kidneys, spleen, and bladder.

Applications: Grind dry cinnamon bark into powder; dissolve 5 g of the powder in warm water, and drink each time, 3 times a day, to cure various types of cold symptoms (including cold abdominal pain, cold abdominal swelling, and cold stomachache).

• Dissolve 5 g of the powder in rice wine, and drink each time, 3 times a day, to alleviate abdominal pain in women after childbirth.

• Dissolve 3 g cinnamon-bark powder in warm water to correct excessive gastric acid and vomiting of acid.

• Use cinnamon bark as a seasoning in cooking to warm up the body.

Experiments: Effects of cinnamon bark on animals indicate it calms the central nervous system in rats and also reduces their blood pressure.

Remarks: As cinnamon has a hot energy, it can treat almost any kind of cold symptoms, and can make the lower region warm (which is good for cold limbs). Some people are fond of cold drinks and cold salads. As time goes on, they may suffer from digestive disorders due to excessive cold energies in the body, which may be treated by cinnamon bark.

• If a woman suffers from irregular periods with post-period pain and whitish vaginal discharge, these are very likely cold symptoms and may be treated by cinnamon bark.

• People at advanced age (65 to 90 years) are usually weak in energy and blood. They have a tendency to develop numbness in their skin and cold arthritis, which means the pain gets worse in cold weather. If this happens, cinnamon bark may be used to correct the conditions.

• Cinnamon bark is such a powerful herb, the Chinese herbalists have listed more than 30 conditions as contraindications of cinnamon bark. Persons with any of these conditions should avoid this herb. The conditions listed as contraindications of cinnamon bark include: hot conditions (including excessive menstrual flow), discharge of urine containing blood, nosebleed, urination difficulty, discharge of dry stools, cough due to hot lungs, fever, loss of voice, hemorrhoids, and other ailments. And anyone suffering from common cold should avoid cinnamon bark. This spice should also be avoided by pregnant women.

• Cinnamon Forests, a city in China named for its ubiquitous cinnamon trees, also has the most beautiful scenic views in the country. When I recently visited Cinnamon Forests I could smell cinnamon everywhere, including the downtown area, and I was pleased as much by the plentiful cinnamon trees in the city as by its beautiful scenery.

Cinnamon Twig (Stick)

Pain in the back and shoulder, chest pain, menopause.

Description: warm; pungent and sweet; induces perspiration, warms the upper region of the body; affects the bladder, heart, lungs.

Applications: Boil 20 g cinnamon twigs with 30 g fresh ginger in enough water to cover the spices; boil until the water is reduced by half. Drink a cupful each time, 3 times a day, to cure arthritis.

• Cook 10 g cinnamon twig with 100 g lean pork in water as a soup; drink it to relieve menopause and excessive gas in the intestine. (Drink the soup as slowly as if consuming liquor.) There is no need to induce perspiration because cinnamon twig is capable of inducing perspiration by itself.

• Boil 3 g cinnamon twigs in water over low heat. Drink it like tea just before bedtime to cure numbness of the skin, fingers, and muscles.

Remarks: Cinnamon twigs are branches from the cinnamon tree. For that reason, the twigs are most effective for arthritis involving the joints of the 4 limbs, because tree branches are comparable to a person's 4 limbs. Many Chinese herbalists describe the functions of cinnamon twigs like streets of a city branching out, with the effects reaching every part of the body. Cinnamon twigs are particularly effective for the symptoms of the limbs and fingers, because fingertips are considered the most remote areas in the human body, beyond the reach of many other herbs.

• Cinnamon twig is basically a warm herb. It can induce perspiration, eliminate cold, promote blood circulation, facilitate menstrual flow, and promote urination. Obviously, this herb is good for rheumatic pain that worsens on exposure to cold, and for cold abdominal pain. But on the other hand, this herb is bad for hot symptoms and ailments, including dry lips, thirst, sore throat, vomiting of blood, fever, ulcers, and alcoholism.

Garlic

Cold abdominal pain, edema, diarrhea, dysentery, whooping cough.

Description: warm; pungent; promotes energy circulation, warms the stomach and spleen, destroys worms; affects the spleen, stomach, and lungs.

Applications: Boil 3 garlic cloves in water and eat with soy sauce at meals to relieve cough and abdominal pain and also to promote blood circulation and urination.

• For women, to relieve itch in the genital region, boil a few garlic cloves and use the liquid to wash the genital region.

• Crush a few garlic cloves to mix with mustard (powder or paste) and eat it with rice wine. Or, boil a few garlic cloves in water and drink it as tea to correct chronic cold sensations, particularly in women. If wine is desired, make garlic wine: Simply cut up a garlic clove in large pieces, drop into a small bottle of wine; put away for 1 month and it is ready to drink as a wine tonic.

• Eat 1 to 3 fresh garlic cloves daily by dividing them into 3 dosages; continue treatment for 5 to 10 consecutive days to heal amebic dysentery.

• Take 2 teaspoonfuls 10 to 20 percent garlic solution every 2 hours (mixed with some syrup or orange tincture to make it more appetizing) to relieve whooping cough in children.

• Eat garlic cloves regularly to prevent bacillary dysentery when it is widespread.

• Cut up a garlic clove and use the juicy slice to rub the skin to relieve pain caused by insect bite (such as bee sting) as an emergency measure.

• Garlic may be cooked with soybeans: Soak the soybeans overnight; cook soybeans with 5 to 10 garlic cloves. Eat as a tonic and also to promote urination, relieve edema, and chronic nephritis.

• Another way to use garlic: Fry garlic cloves in vegetable oil with black pepper, sliced fresh ginger, and salt; add dry shrimps, then sprinkle with sugar, vinegar and green onion. Add some tomato ketchup and flour to thicken, if desired. This recipe contains almost all the needed flavors—sweet, sour, pungent, and salty.

Clinical report: For treatment of lobar pneumonia; 1 tablespoon garlic syrup every 4 hours (in general 10 percent, but sometimes 100 percent). Among the 9 people treated, 6 cases show complete recovery, 3 show no satisfactory results.

Remarks: There have been fewer cases of pulmonary tuberculosis in Sandong, a province of China where people consume more garlic than in any other province. As a result of these findings, garlic has been made into tablets and used with good results.

In the northern provinces of China, Chinese people carry some garlic with them while on a long journey, just in case they have to drink water from mountains or rivers. To prevent bad effects, they chew a garlic clove like chewing gum and spit it out before drinking water.

• Many people don't want to eat garlic for fear of getting bad breath. According to some people, "garlic" breath can be eliminated by eating a few red dates or a persimmon. When garlic cloves are steamed (over boiling water), the strong smell will be gone before eating the garlic.

• In daily cooking, a few garlic slices may be added to eliminate the strong smell of meats or fish. It is believed that a small quantity of garlic can counteract cancer, but an excessive quantity of garlic can cause cancer (based on the Chinese theory that excessive garlic is bad for the stomach and liver).

• Chinese people eat large quantities of garlic only under special circumstances, such as severe malnutrition or edema.

• In recent years, garlic has emerged as an important ingredient in Chinese medicine, mostly due to its powerful effects in treating dysentery and destroying germs. In fact, many modern medicines contain garlic as an important ingredient. For dysentery at its early stage, chew a garlic clove five or six times a day every four hours.

• Contraindications of garlic include eye diseases and sore throat.

Clove

Vomiting, hiccuping, upset stomach, diarrhea, abdominal pain, hernia.

Description: warm; pungent; pushes downward, warms internal region in general and kidneys in particular; affects the stomach, spleen, and kidneys.

Applications: Chew 1 or 2 cloves to get rid of bad breath.

• Apply ground cloves to nipples to heal cracked nipples.

• Grind cloves and persimmon calynx into powder; take 2 g each time in water, twice a day, to relieve hiccupping.

• Boil 4 g cloves with 6 g persimmon calyx, and 4 g fresh ginger in 2 cups water over low heat until water is reduced to 1 cup; drink half a cupful each time, twice a day, to stop vomiting.

• A traditional Chinese formula to relieve hiccupping: Combine 2 g cloves, 3 g persimmon calyx (available in most Chinese herb shops), 3 g ginseng, and 2 g dried ginger and boil; divide into 2 dosages and drink in 1 day. In my experience, this has never failed to produce instant results.

• Boil 20 cloves with red tea leaves and enough water to cover; drink it as tea to correct poor appetite and discomfort in the stomach from indigestion and also to correct excessive gastric acid.

Remarks: Clove is a very warm spice, and as such can warm the stomach and relieve vomiting, hiccupping and hernia pain. But sometimes vomiting and hiccupping are due to hot energy and clove should not be used. If you develop hiccupping and take clove for relief, normally it will take effect in a few minutes, or at most, a few hours. But if clove does not relieve the symptoms, then most probably, they are hot symptoms. Most symptoms of vomiting and hiccupping are cold symptoms, however, and clove may be used for relief.

Fresh Ginger

Common cold, vomiting, cough, asthma, diarrhea.

Description: warm; pungent; induces perspiration, disperses cold, and relieves vomiting; affects the lungs, stomach, and spleen.

Applications: Grate fresh old ginger (see Remarks below) and boil in water for 10 minutes; drink it like tea to cure edema or vomiting or cough and also to warm up the body.

• Crush 100 g fresh old ginger and boil it; use the hot liquid to wash the body and stimulate the skin to induce perspiration for relief of fever in common cold.

• Grate fresh old ginger and squeeze the juice; mix the juice with sugar or honey in 1 to 2 cups boiling water; drink a cupful each time, 3 times a day, to relieve cough.

• Eat a few pieces tender, fresh ginger to relieve indigestion.

• Squeeze fresh ginger juice and drink it as orange juice to heal motion sickness, hiccup, or vomiting; it is also effective to counteract food poisoning.

• Boil 2 g dried ginger or 7 g fresh ginger with some brown sugar and drink it hot to relieve discomfort of cold and fever with cold abdominal pain due to common cold.

• Boil 4 g fresh ginger with 8 g dried orange peel and drink it like tea to heal vomiting and cough due to common cold.

• Western doctors normally use ginger as a digestive and carminative.

Clinical reports: Injection of 5 to 10 percent fresh ginger juice into the affected areas is effective to relieve rheumatic pain.

• Mix 50 g fresh ginger with 30 g brown sugar; to treat acute bacillary dysentery, eat 3 times a day, for 7 days as a treatment program. Among the 50 cases treated, 70 percent recover from the disease and 30 percent show improvements. After eating the ginger mixture, abdominal pain and tenesmus disappear within an average of 1 and 5 days respectively. Stools and bowel movements return to normal within an average of 4 and 5 days respectively.

Remarks: In everyday cooking, fresh tender ginger is used; but when used for therapeutic purposes, fresh old ginger gives better effects. (Fresh ginger, also called "baby" ginger, is available in Chinese shops seasonally, usually in June and July and can be used to make ginger pickle; old ginger, known as "mother" ginger, is difficult to chew and usually available in Chinese markets.)
• Like garlic, ginger is widely used in cooking; a few slices added to cooking will counteract the strong smell of meats, fish, or shellfish and it can also counteract toxic effects.

Dried Ginger

Cold abdominal pain, vomiting and diarrhea, cold limbs, rheumatism.

Description: hot; pungent; warms the internal region; affects the spleen, stomach, and lungs.
Application: Dissolve 7 g dried ground ginger in warm water and drink each time, once a day, to relieve diarrhea with discharge of very watery stools.
Remarks: Dried ginger, available in herb shops, is normally used as herb; when fresh old ginger is peeled and put under the sun to dry, it becomes dried ginger with a hot energy instead of a warm energy.

Nutmeg

Abdominal swelling and pain, diarrhea, vomiting, indigestion.

Description: warm; pungent; pushes downwards; warms the internal region; promotes digestion; affects the spleen and large intestine.
Remarks: Nutmeg is bad for hemorrhoids, hot diarrhea, and toothache. Mace, the spice ground from the layer between the nutmeg shell and its outer husk, is used as a carminative, stomachic tonic, and stimulant.

Marjoram

Common colds, fever, vomiting, diarrhea, jaundice,
malnutrition in children, skin rash.

Description: cool; pungent; induces perspiration; promotes energy circulation; relieves water retention.
Applications: Boil marjoram in water and drink it like tea to induce perspiration.
• Boil marjoram in water and use the liquid to wash the mouth to counteract bad breath.
• To relieve itch, boil 150 g fresh marjoram and use the liquid to wash the affected region.

Experiments: Marjoram promotes urination, induces perspiration, increases the appetite, and also relieves mucous discharge, experiments show.

Remarks: In Chinese folk medicine, marjoram is believed to regulate body temperature and prevent hot diseases; it is widely used in summer as substitute for tea.

Chinese Parsley (Coriander)

Indigestion, measles prior to the rash.

Description: warm; pungent; induces perspiration, promotes digestion, speeds the outbreak of measles rash; affects the lungs and spleen.

Applications: Boil Chinese parsley with water chestnut and carrot to make soup to facilitate eruptions in measles; or, cut up a few whole parsleys (including leaves and roots) and cook in water; wash the measles patient while the liquid is warm to facilitate measles eruptions.

• Regular consumption of Chinese parsley will reduce the bad smell of urine due to internal heat.

• Cook whole Chinese parsley (including leaves and roots) with fish, pork, or beef to remove offensive smells (including vaginal odors and bad breath).

• Use Chinese parsley as a seasoning in cooking to relieve excessive gastric acid and cold stomachache.

Remarks: Chinese people use Chinese parsley as a seasoning when cooking shrimps, crabs, oysters, clams, and other fish for 3 purposes: To make the food look better, to increase the aromatic fragrance, and to increase the warm energy.

• When Chinese parsley is used to facilitate eruptions in measles, a number of things should be kept in mind: Chinese parsley is not intended for prolonged consumption; when there are signs of eruptions on the second or third day of fever in measles, it is the best time to administer Chinese parsley. But if eruptions have already occurred, Chinese parsley should not be used, because it may increase the internal heat.

• People with constant thirst or cracked lips or constipation should not eat Chinese parsley.

Black and White Pepper

Cold abdominal pain, upset stomach, vomiting of clear water, diarrhea, food poisoning.

Description: hot; pungent; pushes downwards; warms the internal regions; affects the stomach and large intestine.

Applications: Boil 30 g sliced fresh ginger with 1 g ground black pepper in 3 cups water until water reduced to 1 cup. Drink this amount 3 times a day for 1 day to stop vomiting due to upset stomach.

Grind 10 black peppercorns into powder and bring to the boil in 8¼ cups water; use the liquid to wash the affected region twice a day to cure eczema of the scrotum.

Experiments: Twenty-four normal adults were given 1 g black pepper to put in their mouths without swallowing it to determine the effects of black pepper on blood pressure and pulse rates. It was found that black pepper can elevate blood pressure: On the average, systolic pressure rises 13.1 mm of mercury; diastolic pressure rises 18.1 mm of mercury; both pressures return to normal in 10 to 15 minutes; no effects were found on pulse rates. During the experiment, the majority of subjects felt hot sensations in their entire bodies or in their heads in addition to the pungent and hot sensations at the tip of their tongues. The effects of black pepper were found to be similar to those of red pepper, only to a lesser degree.

Clinical reports: A report on simple indigestive diarrhea: grind 1 g white pepper into powder and mix with 9 g glucose powder in water; children less than a year old take .3 to .5 g each time; children less than 3 years take .5 to 1.5 g, normally not exceeding 2 g, 3 times a day for 1 to 3 days as a treatment program; in case of dehydration, fluid retention therapy should be applied. Among the 20 cases of simple indigestive diarrhea treated, 18 cases recovered and 2 cases showed improvements.

• A report on nephritis: Make a hole in a chicken egg and squeeze 7 white peppercorns into the egg; seal the hole with flour. Wrap the egg with a wet sheet of paper; steam the egg until cooked. Peel the egg and eat it with the peppercorns. As a treatment program, adults eat 2 eggs a day and children eat 1 egg a day for 10 days. The second program begins 3 days after completing the first program. Generally, 3 treatment programs are administered. Among the 6 cases of nephritis treated, all recovered except a case of chronic nephritis with a ten-year history.

Remarks: Traditionally, black and white peppers are considered useful in warming the body and eliminating the strong smell of meats and fish. But an excessive consumption of these spices is considered harmful and not recommended for people with eye diseases and sore throat.

Red or Green Pepper

Abdominal pain, vomiting, diarrhea.

Description: hot; pungent; warms the internal region, increases appetite, promotes digestion; affects the heart and spleen.

Applications: Red pepper may be used in cooking to excite the spirits, induce

perspiration, promote urination, increase appetite, and soften up blood vessels. Some people believe that red pepper can prevent heart disease.
• Cook red pepper leaves with chicken egg and fresh ginger as a soup to warm up the stomach.
• Use red pepper as a seasoning in cooking to promote blood circulation and also to soften up blood vessels (good for relief of arteriosclerosis and for prevention of hypertension).
Remarks: Consumption of red pepper in excessive quantitites will cause abdominal pain and constipation: Red pepper is not recommended for people with eye disease, cough, gastritis, or nephritis.
• In addition to the color of peppers (which may be red or green), there are also different degrees of intensity: Peppers with a round shape are not as hot as peppers that are long and pointed.
• It is said that there are 4 stages in the psychology of eating red or green pepper: At the beginning, before one starts eating it, one is afraid of its hot nature; gradually, one can tolerate its hot nature; and then, one is used to it and no longer afraid of its hot nature; and finally, one starts complaining that it is not hot enough any more.

Caraway Seed

Stomachache, abdominal pain, hernia, lumbago.

Description: warm; slightly pungent; promotes energy circulation; good for the stomach; affects the kidneys and stomach.
Applications: Boil 10 g caraway seed with 5 g cinnamon and 5 g dried ginger; drink it as soup to treat vomiting and hiccupping.
• Boil 10 g fennel seed in 3 cups water over low heat until water is reduced to 1 cup. Drink a cupful each time, twice a day, to relieve cough.
Experiment: Caraway has been found to relieve asthma in rats.
Remarks: Basically, the actions of caraway are similar to fennel.

Peppermint

Common cold, headache, sore throat, indigestion, canker, toothache, skin eruptions.

Description: cool; pungent; affects the lungs and liver.
Applications: Boil 5 g peppermint in 1 cup water for a short while. Drink it as tea to treat discharge of stools containing blood (as in dysentery).

• Squeeze fresh peppermint juice for use as ear drops to relieve earache. (To squeeze the juice, use a pestle to pound the peppermint lightly, then wrap in a clean cloth and squeeze out the juice; or wrap peppermint, pound it and squeeze.)

• Boil 5 g fresh peppermint in 1 cup water and add a little salt. Drink it like tea to relieve all kinds of pain involving the head and neck, such as headache, sore throat, pain in the mouth, pain in the tongue, toothache, and also nosebleed, preferably at the early stage.

• Cook 70 g fresh peppermint with 150 g pork liver; eat it at meals to relieve pain in the eye, blurred vision, and watering of the eyes.

• Boil fresh peppermint with bean curd and fresh ginger in water. Drink the soup and eat the bean curd to heal nasal congestion and nasal discharge, frequent sneezing, and common cold.

Experiment: Local applications of menthol (a type of peppermint oil) are effective for headache, neuralgia, and itching. When menthol is used, the skin feels cool sensations followed by light burning sensations. The cool sensations induced by menthol are not caused by a lowering of skin temperature but rather by the cold receptor of the nerve endings.

Remarks: If skin itchiness is due to cold skin, menthol will make it worse; normally, when skin itchiness occurs in winter or on exposure to cold weather, it means that the person has a cold skin.

• Peppermint can cure trigeminal neuralgia and I have a personal experience in this respect. About 10 years ago, I had developed trigeminal neuralgia, which was very painful, and I had used peppermint for instant relief of pain. It was more effective than any pain killer. But treatment of trigeminal neuralgia must be based upon each person's physical constitution.

Spearmint

Common cold, cough, headache, abdominal pain, menstrual pain.

Description: warm; pungent and sweet; promotes energy circulation, relieves pain.

Applications: Cook tender, fresh peppermint leaves in water with chicken egg and eat as soup to treat headache.

• Spearmint calms down the spirits and relieves common cold at the same time. It has been used in Chinese folk medicine to treat headache and dizziness. It is reported that a woman was suffering from chronic headache for a decade, particularly when she was under stress, with headache attacks, sometimes many times a day. Her malady was diagnosed by Western doctors as a case of cerebral anemia and by traditional Chinese doctors as something else, but no relief was offered. She eventually healed herself by drinking spearmint soup for less than 1 month.

• It is believed that Vietnamese women regard spearmint as an important herb for relief of headache; they just drink it as tea.

Remarks: Spearmint could be effective for relief of headache because it can act upon the liver, and in Chinese medicine the liver is responsible for headache due to stress.

Ginseng

Poor appetite, fatigue, upset stomach, diarrhea, cough, excessive perspiration, forgetfulness, impotence, frequent urination, diabetes, vaginal bleeding.

Description: warm; sweet, and slightly bitter; tones up energy; produces fluids; calms the spirits; affects the spleen and lungs.

Applications: Ginseng is one of the few Chinese herbs that is frequently applied alone. A traditional Chinese herbal formula—solitary ginseng soup—is made by steaming or boiling ginseng for consumption: Boil 5 g ginseng in 1½ cups water over low heat until water is reduced to half. Drink it all within 1 day to cure prolapse and heart failure.

• Ginseng may be used with dry ginger to treat morning sickness and abdominal pain.

Remarks: Ginseng is regarded as an important ingredient to perform the following groups of functions:

• To excite the nervous system, improve working efficiency, and reduce fatigue.

• To stimulate blood forming organs and aid the blood production.

• To increase the heart's contraction capacity and to tone up the heart (useful in the treatment of heart failure and shock).

• To improve the sex gland functions in men and women in the treatment of hypogonadism.

• To improve the functions of digestion, absorption, and metabolism.

• To act as an antidiuretic.

• To lower blood sugar; this function is attributed to the presence of ginsenin in ginseng.

While ginseng has its important functions, there are also circumstances under which ginseng should not be used. Such circumstances may include the following:

• Cough and coughing up blood. Vomiting of blood due to excessive indulgence in sexual intercourse.

• Ginseng could cause encephalemia or cerebrovascular accidents in people suffering from hypertension.

• Edema and incomplete functions of the kidneys with decreased urination, because ginseng is an antidiuretic that may cause edema to deteriorate.
• Excessive type of insomnia, because ginseng can make an excessive condition even more excessive.
• Common cold with fever, because ginseng can increase the production of extreme heat in the body, which can intensify the fever.

There are three basic kinds of ginseng with different functions: Chinese ginseng; Korean or red ginseng, and American ginseng. Chinese ginseng, more beneficial to the lungs and the digestive system, is more often used to benefit the lungs, produce fluids, and heal other critical symptoms. Korean or red ginseng is warmer; it is most frequently used to tone up energy and blood to improve the functions of the sex gland and is less effective for other symptoms. American ginseng has a cool energy. It tastes sweet and slightly bitter, acting on the heart, the lungs, and the kidneys, and is mostly used for cough, thirst, and alcoholism.

Rosemary

Headache.

Description: warm; pungent; induces perspiration; used as a stomachic.
Remarks: One source indicates that rosemary preparation can be used as an emmenagogue to speed up menstrual flow in menopause syndrome. Another source indicates that rosemary oil and hollylock root mixtures can promote growth of hair on head. Still another source indicates that infusions of rosemary and borax can prevent baldness.

Saffron

Congested chest, vomiting of blood, suppression of menstruation, abdominal pain after childbirth due to blood coagulations, injuries from falls.

Description: neutral; sweet; promotes energy and blood circulation, eliminates blood coagulations; affects the heart and liver.
Experiments: On animals, an experiment shows that saffron can induce tensions and contractions of the uterus with signs of excitation. Another experiment on cats shows the effect of saffron in lowering blood pressure. A third experiment on rats shows the effect of saffron in prolonging their estrous cycle from 1 or 2 to 3 or 4 days.
Remarks: Saffron styles, stigmas, and flowers are used by Chinese people for therapies.

Thyme

Whooping cough, acute bronchitis, laryngitis.

Description: suppresses cough; also used as an aromatic calmative.
Experiments: Thyme can be used as an antibacterial agent and an anthelmintic. Thyme leaf may be used as an expectorant, according to experiments.

Licorice

Abdominal pain, poor appetite, fatigue, fever, cough, palpitations, convulsions, sore throat, digestive ulcers, drug poisoning, food poisoning.

Description: neutral; sweet; slows down acute diseases, lubricates lungs, counteracts toxic effects, coordinates the effects of other herbs; affects the spleen, stomach, and lungs.
Applications: Prepare 150 g processed licorice and 80 g dry ginger; boil in only enough water to cover the 2 ingredients; boil until the water is reduced by half; strain and drink 1 cup of the warm soup each time, twice a day, to cure abscessed lungs, suppurative pneumonia, and bronchitis without cough.
• Boil 10 g licorice with 20 g whole wheat kernels and 5 Chinese red dates. Drink as soup to treat hysteria in women, anxiety, and stress. This is a time-honored herbal formula in Chinese medicine.
Remarks: Licorice is a very important herb in Chinese medicine. There are 2 kinds: raw licorice and licorice processed with honey. Raw licorice is slightly cool and tastes sweet, which can relieve hot symptoms and counteract toxic effects. Processed licorice is slightly warm and tastes sweet, which can tone up the spleen and increase energy.

5
Fruits and Nuts

Apple

Indigestion, low blood sugar, morning sickness, chronic enteritis.

Description: cool; sweet and sour; produces fluids; lubricates the lungs; promotes digestion; relieves intoxication.

Applications: Peel and core a few half-ripe apples and press or crush them to squeeze out the juice. Drink half a cup of juice each time, 3 times a day for 3 consecutive days, to remedy indigestion.

• Eat 2 peeled apples each time, twice a day for 3 consecutive days as a treatment program to treat low blood sugar.

• Prepare 6 fresh apples: Peel, core and remove seeds; crush apples and steam them with 500 g honey until as soft as jelly. Take 2 teaspoonfuls each time, 3 times a day, to treat cough due to hot lungs and dry sensations in the mouth and tongue. This remedy is also good for neutralizing the effects of smoking.

• Prepare 30 to 60 g fresh apple peel. Fry 30 g rice until yellowish; mix the rice with apple peel to make tea to alleviate morning sickness.

• Cut a few unripe apples into 4 slices; dry the slices in the sun; grind into powder. Take 15 g apple powder with 1 cup warm water, twice a day, to cure chronic enteritis, abdominal pain, and diarrhea.

Banana

Constipation, hemorrhoids, hypertension, alcoholism.

Description: cold; sweet; lubricates the intestines; detoxicates.

Applications: Eat 1 to 2 very soft bananas twice a day before bedtime and first thing in the morning on an empty stomach to relieve constipation.

• Eat 1 to 2 fresh bananas, three times a day, to relieve thirst in a hot disease.

• Steam 2 half-ripe bananas with their peels until very soft. Eat twice a day, the first thing in the morning on an empty stomach and before bedtime, to

cure hemorrhoids and discharge of blood from anus after bowel movements.
• Boil 1 banana peel or stem in water, and drink it as tea, a cupful each time, 3 times a day, to treat and prevent hypertension.
• Place 500 g banana and 15 g black sesame in a blender and mix them. Eat in one day to treat hypertension with constipation.
• Steam 2 very soft bananas with their peels. Eat the banana and peel twice a day, first thing in the morning on an empty stomach and before bedtime, to cure asthma and cough due to hot lungs.
• Boil 60 g banana peel in water and drink the liquid for relief of alcoholism and hangover.
Experiment: An experiment on animals shows unripe banana is effective in the treatment and prevention of gastric ulcers.

Cherry

Paralysis, numbness of arms and legs, rheumatism, lumbago, frostbite.

Description: warm; sweet.
Applications: Chew 8 to 12 fresh cherries slowly like chewing gum, twice a day, to relieve pharyngolaryngitis at its early stage.
• Boil 1 K fresh cherries until very soft; remove and discard seeds. Add 500 g sugar and boil to make jelly. Take a spoonful cherry jelly each time, twice a day, to relieve fatigue and improve your complexion.
• In a large jar, combine 500 g fresh cherries and 4½ cups rice wine; cover and store for 10 days. Drink 30 to 60 g cherry wine each time, twice a day, to alleviate numbness of joints and paralysis from rheumatism.
Remarks: Cherries are not recommended for people with internal heat because they generate heat in the body. Therefore, cherries are recommended for the cold type of arthritis and rheumatism.

Cherry Seed

Measles, sty in the eyelid, scar.

Description: neutral; bitter and pungent; helps promote outbreak of rash in measles; counteracts toxic effects.
Applications: Grind cherry seeds into powder and mix with water for external application to the affected region to cure a sty.
• Boil cherry seeds in water; use the liquid to wash the affected skin to eliminate a scar.
• Boil 9 g cherry seeds in 1 cup water and drink the liquid to promote outbreak

of rash in measles. In addition, boil 150 g cherry seeds in 4 cups water; wash the body with the liquid.

• Crush 90 to 150 g cherry seeds with a pestle or hammer and boil in water. Wash the affected skin with the liquid to heal a carbuncle.

Coconut

Tapeworm and fasciolopsiasis, edema, vomiting, constipation, premature aging.

Description: warm (liquid inside coconut and shell); neutral and obstructive (shell); slightly sweet and aromatic (liquid); sweet (coconut meat); the liquid and coconut meat produce fluids, promote urination, and destroy intestinal worms; the shell constricts and destroys intestinal worms and relieves itching.

Applications: Drink coconut liquid to relieve thirst, sunstroke, fever, diabetes, edema.

• Drink a glass of coconut liquid with 30 g sugar and a little salt, 3 times a day for 3 consecutive days, and then once a day afterwards, to relieve vomiting and weakness after severe bleeding and dehydration after severe diarrhea.

• Consume coconut meat and coconut liquid once a day, first thing in the morning on an empty stomach for 3 consecutive days, to relieve tapeworm and fasciolopsiasis.

• Eat meat of 1 coconut each time, in the morning and evening, to correct constipation.

• Cut the meat of a coconut into small cubes and mix with sugar. Put the coconut cubes in a jar; cover with sugar and store for 2 weeks. Eat 2 to 3 coconut sugar cubes each time, twice a day, to tone up weakness in the elderly and prevent premature aging.

Fig

Enteritis, dysentery, constipation, hemorrhoids, sore throat, diarrhea.

Description: neutral; sweet; detoxicates; used as stomachic tonic; affects the spleen and large intestine.

Applications: Eat 1 to 2 fresh figs each time, in the morning and evening, to wake up appetite and correct indigestion.

• Eat 1 to 2 fresh figs at bedtime to relieve constipation, particularly in the elderly.

• Steam until very soft 1 to 2 fresh figs and 2 honey dates (processed in honey). Eat 1 to 2 figs each day to relieve dry cough and sore throat.

• Boil 1 kg dry figs in water at low heat until they are soft as jelly. Add

750 g sugar and heat until sugar dissolves. Then mix all the ingredients; take 1 teaspoonful fig jelly each time, in the morning and evening, to correct weakness after illness. Fig jelly is also used as adjuvant therapy for pulmonary tuberculosis and hepatitis.

• Boil until very soft 1 to 3 fresh figs or 30 g dry figs with 60 g lean pork and 2 red dates; eat once a day to increase milk secretion in women after childbirth.

• Boil 60 g fresh figs with 60 g pork or with 1 chicken egg and 15 g rice wine. Eat once a day to relieve pain in muscles and bones, and numbness from rheumatism.

• Fry 30 g dry figs until aromatic; separately, fry 9 g dry ginger until it looks like charcoal. Boil together the figs and ginger. Eat 3 times a day, to cure chronic diarrhea.

• Eat 2 unripe fresh figs in the morning and evening to alleviate pain and bleeding in hemorrhoids.

Remarks: Fig leaf is neutral in energy and tastes sweet and slightly pungent; it can heal hemorrhoids and heart pain and swelling.

Fig Root

Pain in muscles and bone, hemorrhoids, tuberculosis of lymph node.

Applications: Boil fresh or dried fig or fig roots in water with pork or eggs for pain in muscles and bones.

• Crush fig roots (with rough surfaces removed); boil in water to make tea to remedy itching in the throat.

• Boil 30 g fig and fig roots to relieve tuberculosis of lymph node.

Grape

Blood and energy deficiency, cough, palpitations, night sweat, rheumatism, difficulty when urinating, edema.

Description: neutral; sweet and sour; strengthens the tendons and bones; promotes urination; also used as blood tonic and energy tonic; affects the lungs, spleen, and kidneys.

Applications: Crush 500 g fresh grapes; add 500 g rice wine and mix thoroughly. Strain to make grape wine. Eat 30 g of the soaked raisins or drink 30 g grape wine in the morning and evening, to tone up energy after illness.

• Eat a large bunch of fresh grapes in the morning and evening, to relieve dry throat and thirst.

• Boil 30 g raisins with 15 g fresh ginger peel. Drink twice a day to cure nutritional edema.

• Squeeze juice from 250 g fresh grapes and mix with an equal amount of

warm water. Drink it all each time, once a day, to relieve pain on urination, difficult urination, and discharge of short and reddish stream of urine.
• Crush 120 g fresh grapes and 250 g fresh lotus roots. Squeeze out the juice, drink it all each time, 3 times a day, to cure or prevent discharge of urine containing blood.
• Boil 30 g raisins in water and drink it like soup. In addition, boil grapevine leaves and parsley and use the liquid to wash the body to promote the outbreak of rash in measles.
• Boil 30 g raisins with 15 g red dates in water; drink like soup to relieve anxiety during quickening.
Remarks: Eating excessive quantities of grapes may decrease appetite.

Guava Leaf

Diarrhea, chronic dysentery, eczema, bleeding due to injuries.

Description: neutral; sweet; obstructive.
Applications: Boil about 50 g fresh guava leaves in water; drink the juice to cure or prevent enteritis, dysentery, and diarrhea.
• Apply fresh guava leaf juice to injuries to stop bleeding.

Grapefruit

*Indigestion, bad breath due to intoxication,
poor appetite in pregnant women.*

Description: cold; sweet and sour.
Applications: Steam 90 g peeled grapefruit with half a cup rice wine and 1 cup honey. Drink it all in 1 day to relieve cough with mucous discharge.
• Eat 1 medium grapefruit each time, 3 times a day, to relieve indigestion, belching, and mouth watering in pregnant women.
• Slowly eat 1 small grapefruit to relieve intoxication.

Grapefruit Peel

Congestion in chest, mucous discharge, cough, intoxication.

Description: warm; pungent, sweet, and bitter; pushes downwards; affects the spleen, kidneys, and bladder.
Applications: Collect grapefruit peels; cut off only the outer rind. Put rinds in the sun to dry to make dry grapefruit peels. Or, instead of drying the peels in the sun, boil the peels in water for a while. Drain and put the peels in the sun to half-dry them; then add sugar to make candied grapefruit peels.

• Chew 30 to 60 g candied grapefruit peels slowly, like chewing gum, to relieve motion sickness and vomiting.
• Boil 15 g candied grapefruit peels or 3 g dry grapefruit peels in water and drink like soup, 3 times a day, to alleviate abdominal swelling and pain and diarrhea caused by indigestion in children.

Guava

Diarrhea, diabetes, hemorrhoids.

Description: warm; sweet; obstructive and constrictive; stops diarrhea and bleeding.
Applications: Crush 250 g fresh guavas and bring to a boil. Drink it all each time, 3 times a day, to relieve diarrhea in acute gastroenteritis and dysentery.
• Fry 30 g dry guavas; boil guavas in water and divide into 3 dosages to drink in 1 day to relieve diarrhea in children.
• Crush 90 g fresh guavas; squeeze out the juice to drink before meals, 3 times a day, to alleviate the symptoms associated with diabetes.
• Boil 90 g dry guavas and drink as tea, to relieve acute and chronic pharyngolaryngitis and hoarseness.
• Boil 500 g fresh guavas or 250 g dry guavas until the liquid becomes very concentrated; use the guava liquid to wash the affected region, 2 to 3 times a day, to remedy hemorrhoids, bleeding, eczema, itching, and heat rash.

Hawthorn Fruit

Meat indigestion, abdominal swelling, mucous discharge, discharge of blood from anus, lumbago, hernia, neck pain after childbirth.

Description: slightly warm; sweet and sour; promotes digestion; corrects blood coagulations; expels tapeworm; affects the spleen, stomach, and liver.
Applications: Soak hawthorn fruit in boiling water for less than 1 minute; slice the fruits and lay them in the sun to dry. (Hawthorn fruit slices are available in most Chinese herb shops.)
• Fry hawthorn slices until they look like charcoal to make hawthorn fruit charcoal.
• Mix together the following ingredients and marinate for 10 days to prepare hawthorn fruit wine: 250 g hawthorn slices, 250 g fresh longans, 30 g red dates, 30 g brown sugar, and 4½ cups rice wine.
• Drink 30 to 60 g hawthorn fruit wine at every bedtime to relieve pain caused by excessive fatigue, muscular pain, and arthritis pain, flying spots in front of the eyes, lumbago and pain in thigh in the elderly.
• Boil in water 60 g hawthorn fruit slices with an equal amount fresh or dried

chestnuts until very soft; add 30 g sugar and stir thoroughly. Drink the juice once a day, first thing in the morning on an empty stomach, to cure scurvy.
• Boil 31 g hawthorn slices with water; stir in 1.5 g fennel powder. Drink the juice in the morning and evening to relieve hernia of the small intestine.
• Boil 15 g hawthorn fruit slices in water and drink as tea on a long-term basis, to relieve hypertension, high level of blood fat, and coronary heart disease.
• Grind 6 to 9 g hawthorn fruit charcoal into powder. Take the powder with warm water, once a day, to relieve abdominal pain caused by acute and chronic gastritis, enteritis, and dysentery.
• Boil 3 g hawthorn charcoal with 6 g hawthorn fruit slices; drink the juice to relieve diarrhea in children; or crush 5 hawthorn fruits and squeeze out the juice to mix with a pinch of hawthorn fruit charcoal for oral administration to stop diarrhea in children.
• Crush 2 to 3 fresh hawthorn fruits and squeeze out the juice to drink; or boil 2 to 3 hawthorn fruits with 6 g dry orange peels; drink the juice to correct indigestion, abdominal swelling, and abdominal pain.
Experiments: An experiment on rabbits shows the effects of hawthorn fruit in lowering blood pressure.
• An experiment on toads shows the effects of hawthorn fruit in expanding blood vessels.
• Hawthorn fruits are reported to have the effects of contracting the uterus and reducing antibiosis.
Remarks: Hawthorn fruits are not recommended for people suffering from constipation due to internal heat or those who have excessive gastric acid.
• Hawthorn fruits can effectively digest fat and prevent it from entering into the blood vessels by removing it through the bowel movements. Indeed, the fruits are so effective in softening hard substances, the Chinese people use it to cook stubborn and tough old chickens! When hawthorn fruits are used in the cooking water, the tough chickens become soft and tender—an indication of the tenderizing power of this fruit. Another example, when hawthorn fruits are used to cook fish, even the fish bones will become tender.

Lemon

Cough with mucous discharge, indigestion, diabetes, pharyngolaryngitis.

Description: extremely sour; produces fluids; secures fetus in quickening, considered good for pregnant women.
Applications: To make preserved lemons, place 500 g fresh lemons in a large earthenware container; add 250 g salt and leave the container in the sun to dry until the peels become wrinkled and soft with the juices flowing out. The

older preserved lemons are the best. Eat preserved lemons with meals to relieve indigestion.

• Peel a lemon and squeeze it to make lemonade for relief of summer heat, diabetes, and pharyngolaryngitis.

• Steam a fresh lemon with an adequate amount of rock sugar. Eat it in the morning and evening to relieve cough with plenty of mucous discharge and whooping cough in children.

Remarks: Lemon is not recommended for people with gastric or duodenal ulcers and excessive gastric acid.

• Lemon seed is neutral and bitter and good to use to stimulate energy and relieve pain.

• Crush 15 g lemon seeds and grind into powder. Dissolve 3 g lemon seed powder in water each time, once a day, for 5 consecutive days, to relieve blurred vision.

• Grind lemon seeds into powder. Dissolve 3 g lemon seed powder in a little rice wine. Drink at bedtime to relieve body pain from excessive fatigue.

Mango

Cough, indigestion, bleeding from gums.

Description: cool; sweet and sour; quenches thirst; strengthens the stomach; relieves vomiting; promotes urination.

Applications: Eat a fresh mango with peel each time, 3 times a day, to relieve cough with mucous discharge and asthma.

• Eat a fresh mango with peel in the morning and evening to relieve indigestion, chest congestion, and abdominal swelling.

• Eat 2 mangoes every day to relieve bleeding from gums.

Remarks: An excessive consumption of mango is reported to have caused nephritis.

• Eating mango after a full meal will cause swelling of the stomach.

• Mango should not be eaten with foods that have a pungent flavor, such as garlic or green onion, as it will cause skin itching and jaundice. One day I intentionally ate 5 large mangoes with a small quantity of green onion, partly to determine the validity of this centuries-old belief and partly to enjoy the taste of mango. I developed severe skin itching within 5 hours, but no sign of jaundice, because it takes longer for a person to develop jaundice.

• Mango kernel is neutral, tastes sweet and bitter, and stimulates energy and relieves pain. To use the mango kernel, dry the large, flat seed first and break it up.

• Crush 15 g mango kernels and 15 g longan seeds; add 5 red dates and boil together in 3 cups water until the water is reduced to 1 cup. Drink 1 cup of juice each time, in the morning and evening, to relieve hernial pain and orchitis.

• Boil 15 g of mango peel with 30 g of mango kernel in the amount of water sufficient to cover the two ingredients; drink two cups of juice each time, once a day, to relieve skin edema.

Olive

Sore throat, coughing up blood, alcoholism, diarrhea.

Description: neutral; sweet and sour; obstructive; affects the lungs and stomach.

Applications: Dry fresh olives in the shade for 1 to 2 days. Put olives in a large earthenware container, add salt, and store for 2 weeks to make preserved olives.

• Remove the seed from a fresh or preserved olive and keep the olive in your mouth to relieve sore throat. Repeat with 1 olive each time, a few times a day.

• Boil 5 fresh pitted olives and a piece of crystallized ginger in water. Drink the juice 3 times a day, to cure dysentery and enteritis.

• Boil 5 fresh pitted olives in water; add 100 g fresh lotus root and lean pork and a little salt. Drink the juice only, once a day, to stop bleeding from hemorrhoids and bleeding from the stomach.

• Mix 5 fresh pitted olives and some rock sugar; steam them for half an hour. Eat the olives to relieve chronic cough.

• Crush 5 to 10 fresh pitted olives; add 35 g sugar and 4 cups water; boil for 10 minutes. Drink the juice, once a day, to relieve alcoholism.

Clinical reports: For treatment of acute bacillary dysentery: Use 100 g fresh olives with seeds and boil in a cup of water over very low heat for 2 to 3 hours until reduced to a half cup; strain. Adults drink a half to 1 tablespoonful each time. Repeat 3 to 4 times until bowel movements return to normal. Treatment stops as soon as the patients have 1 to 2 bowel movements daily. In general, each treatment program continues for 5 days.

Tangerine

Chest congestion, vomiting, hiccupping.

Description: cool; sweet and sour; promotes energy circulation; strengthens the spleen; relieves coughing; affects the lungs, stomach, and kidneys.

Applications: Eat a half-ripe tangerine to relieve indigestion and help your digestion.

• Drink fresh tangerine juice to relieve thirst from fever and dry throat, and to relieve a hangover.

• Steam 2 unpeeled tangerines with 30 g rock sugar; eat the tangerines at bedtime to relieve cough with yellowish mucous discharge.

Remarks: Dried tangerine peels can be made by putting tangerine peels in the sun to dry. Dried tangerine peels have a warm energy and pungent-bitter flavor.

• Boil 6 g dried tangerine peels with 3 g fresh ginger in water; drink a cup of the juice each time, twice a day, to relieve vomiting.

• Spread fresh tangerines in the sun until half dry. Press to flatten them; soak the flat tangerines in syrup to make tangerine cakes.

• Chew 1 small tangerine cake slowly, like chewing gum, to relieve vomiting and diarrhea; repeat 4 hours later.

• Tangerine seeds have a neutral energy and bitter flavor.

• To relieve pain and swelling in mastitis, boil 15 g tangerine seeds in a mixture of half water and half wine. Drink a cup of the juice each time, 3 times a day.

• Fry until yellowish 30 g tangerine seeds and grind them; mix the powder with a quarter cup rice wine. Drink the juice twice a day to relieve hernial pain, swelling and pain in testes, and lumbago.

• Fresh tangerine is not recommended for people with a cough from common cold and edema. Tangerine peel is not recommended for anyone with a dry cough or who is vomiting blood.

Mandarin Orange

Thirst, intoxication, urination difficulty, emphysema.

Description: cool; sweet and sour; promotes urination; lubricates the lungs; relieves cough; eliminates mucus.

Applications: Eat a few fresh mandarin oranges to relieve thirst from a fever or painful urination. Repeat 4 hours later.

• Steam a fresh unpeeled mandarin orange with 15 g rock sugar and 2 fresh ginger slices for 1 hour. Eat the orange with peel to treat senile and chronic cough.

• Drink fresh mandarin orange juice to relieve a hangover.

• Steam a fresh unpeeled mandarin orange with 5 red dates for half an hour. Eat the orange and dates to relieve symptoms of emphysema.

• Slowly chew the peel of a fresh mandarin orange to relieve chest congestion and abdominal swelling due to indigestion.

• Mandarin orange seeds may be left in the sun to dry for use in remedies.

• Fry 30 g mandarin orange seeds; boil the seeds in 3 cups water with 9 g caraway seeds until the water is reduced to 2 cups. Drink 1 cup of the juice each time, in the morning and evening, to cure hernia and painful swelling in the testes.

• Crush 15 g mandarin orange seeds and boil them in 30 g rice wine. Drink the juice twice a day to promote milk secretion and to soften a lump in breast.
• Collect mandarin orange peels and dry them in the sun to make dried mandarin orange peels.

Dried Mandarin Orange Peel

Chest congestion, abdominal swelling, lack of appetite, vomiting, hiccupping, coughing with mucous discharge, fish and crab poisoning.

Description: warm; pungent and bitter; pushes downwards; stimulates energy; relieves water retention; eliminates mucus; affects the spleen and lungs.
Applications: Dried mandarin orange peel is an important Chinese herb. It is widely used in remedies.
• Dissolve 1.5 g dry mandarin orange peel powder in warm water. Drink each time, 3 times a day, to relieve chest congestion and abdominal swelling and pain due to indigestion.
• Mix 40 g dry mandarin orange peel powder with 100 g cuttlefish bone powder. Take 3 g dissolved in warm water each time, 3 times a day, to treat stomachache, swelling of stomach, belching, and excessive gastric acid.
Clinical report: For treatment of acute mastitis: Mix 40 g dried mandarin orange peels and 7 g licorice in water. Bring to a boil and then boil it again for a second time. Divide into 2 dosages to take in 1 day. Double the dosage in severe cases. Clinical observations show that early treatment (within 1 to 2 days of onset) produces good results with a 70 percent success rate in 2 to 3 days. This treatment is less effective when acute mastitis has a longer duration. No results are obtained after suppuration has occurred.

Kumquat

Chest congestion, thirst, indigestion, cough, whooping cough, stomachache, hernial pain, poor appetite.

Description: warm; pungent, sweet and sour; relieves cough; eliminates mucus; promotes energy circulation.
Applications: Steam 5 to 10 fresh kumquats with 30 g of rock sugar for half an hour and eat a few each time, twice a day, to stop senile cough and asthma.
• Eat a few fresh kumquats to relieve indigestion.
• To make dried kumquats, place fresh kumquats in the sun to dry.
• Boil 10 dried kumquats in 6 cups water until water is reduced to 3 cups; drink 1 cup of the juice each time, 3 times a day, to treat stomachache.
• Crush 10 dried kumquats and boil in a mixture of half water and half rice

wine. Drink a cup of the juice each time, twice a day, to relieve hernial pain.
• To make sugar kumquats, place fresh kumquats in the sun until half dry. Soak kumquats in syrup.
• Chew 30 g sugar kumquats slowly, like chewing gum, to stimulate poor appetite due to common cold or motion sickness.

Papaya

Stomachache, dysentery, difficulty in bowel movements, rheumatism.

Description: neutral; sweet; promotes digestion; destroys intestinal worms.
Applications: Boil 500 g partially ripe papayas with 2 pork forelegs until very soft. Eat papayas and pork once each day for 3 consecutive days to stimulate lactation after childbirth.
• Steam 250 to 500 g fresh papayas. Eat papayas once a day to relieve thirst from fever and chronic cough.
• Prepare a few unripe papayas: peel and remove seeds; soak papayas in vinegar to make sour papayas (save the soaking vinegar).
• Eat 30 g sour papaya or 60 g fresh papaya twice a day to relieve indigestion and abdominal pain and swelling.
• At bedtime, eat 250 g sour papayas and drink 60 g of the vinegar in which papayas have been soaked, for 3 consecutive days, to destroy tapeworms, roundworms, and whipworms, and other worms of the intestinal tract.
Remarks: Papaya is reported to be antitumorigenic because it contains carpaine.
• It is reported that papaya has a paralytic effect on the central nervous system, which may explain why papaya can relieve rheumatic pain.

Peach

Cough, hernial pain, excessive perspiration.

Description: warm; sweet and sour; obstructive; promotes blood circulation; lubricates the intestines; produces fluids; checks perspiration.
Applications: Peel 3 fresh peaches and steam the peaches with 30 g rock sugar. Eat once a day to treat asthma and cough.
• Fresh unripe peaches may be left in the sun to dry to make dried peaches.
• Boil 30 g dried peaches and a mango in water. Eat twice a day to relieve hernial pain.
• Fry 30 g dried peaches until the surface is brown and yellowish. Add water immediately and then add 30 g red dates; boil for a few minutes. Eat at bedtime to relieve seminal emission, excessive perspiration, and night sweat.
• Eat 1 to 2 peaches each time, twice a day, or boil 30 g dried peaches in water and drink like tea to treat hypertension.

• Break peach seeds to obtain the kernels; leave them in the sun to dry. Peach kernels are important and widely used in Chinese herbal remedies. The kernels have a neutral energy and bittersweet flavor. They are considered slightly toxic and capable of promoting blood circulation and lubricating the intestines.
• Crush 15 g peach kernels and boil with 30 g honey. Drink it to cure constipation.
• Boil 15 g each of peach kernels, fresh ginger, and red dates with 30 g rice wine and an adequate amount of water. Drink as tea in the morning and evening to relieve abdominal pain after childbirth and suppression of menstruation.

Pear

Cough with mucus, constipation, difficulty when swallowing, alcoholism, difficult urination, indigestion.

Description: cool; sweet and slightly sour; produces fluids; lubricates dryness; eliminates mucus; affects the lungs and stomach.
Applications: Drink a glass of fresh pear juice in the morning and evening to relieve cough and thirst from fever.
• Soak fresh unpeeled pears in vinegar to make vinegar pears.
• Peel 2 vinegar pears and eat them to relieve indigestion and alcoholism.
• Crush 2 vinegar pears to squeeze out the juice. Drink the juice slowly in the morning and evening to cure sore throat and difficulty when swallowing.
• Boil 60 g dried pear peels in water. Drink the juice to relieve difficult urination and pain when urinating.

Persimmon

Coughing, vomiting of blood, mouth canker, stomachache, diarrhea, hemorrhoids, hypertension, endemic goitre, discharge of urine containing blood, hiccupping.

Description: cold; sweet; obstructive; quenches thirst; lubricates the lungs; strengthens the spleen; affects the heart, lungs, and large intestine.
Applications: Eat a fresh persimmon, peeled, each time, twice a day, to relieve stomachache that gets worse on exposure to heat.
• Crush a partially ripe persimmon and squeeze out the juice. Drink the juice with warm water once a day to treat hypertension and endemic goitre.
• Pick persimmons when the outer layers just begin to turn yellow; peel persimmons and leave them in the sun on hot days and frequently apply pressure to flatten them until the surface appears coated with white powder.

In the Chinese language, the powder is called white frost of persimmon. Persimmons dried in this manner are called persimmon cakes.

• Steam 2 persimmon cakes with 30 g honey. Eat in the morning and evening to treat senile asthma and cough with mucus.

• Cook 2 persimmon cakes in water with 60 g glutinous (sweet) rice and 2 slices dried orange peel. Eat with meals, once a day for 3 consecutive days, to cure chronic enteritis and diarrhea.

• Mix a persimmon cake with a little long-grain rice and water and crush them to make a paste. Use to feed children 3 times a day for 2 to 3 consecutive days to relieve diarrhea.

• Boil 2 persimmon cakes until very soft. Eat 2 persimmon cakes each time, twice a day, to cure hemorrhoids.

• Cook rice soup and add 2 persimmon cakes to the soup. Eat once a day for 5 consecutive days to relieve discharge of urine containing blood with no pain on urination.

• Crush 3 to 9 g white frost of persimmon; boil in water and drink it slowly, a few times each day, to cure mouth canker, sore throat, and dry cough.

• Gather the calyx and receptacle of a persimmon and leave in the sun to dry. The dried calyx and receptacle, important in Chinese herbal remedies, have a neutral energy, obstructive power, and have the effect of pushing downwards.

• Boil 3 persimmon cakes in water with the calyxes and receptacles until soft. Drink the juice in the morning and evening to treat cough and chest pain in lung disease.

• Boil 9 g calyxes and receptacles in water with 3 g fresh ginger. Drink like tea to relieve hiccupping; or fry 3 g persimmon calyxes and receptacles until aromatic and grind into powder. Dissolve in rice wine and drink once a day to relieve hiccupping.

Pineapple

Edema, indigestion, diarrhea, vomiting, abdominal swelling.

Description: neutral; sweet and sour; promotes urination and digestion; quenches thirst; heals swelling.

Applications: Fry 250 g fresh pineapple, sliced, with 60 g chicken in oil, seasoned with pepper and salt. Eat every day, or every other day, to relieve dizziness due to low blood pressure.

• Eat 4 slices fresh pineapple or drink a glass of fresh pineapple juice each time, twice a day, to relieve indigestion, abdominal swelling, vomiting, or diarrhea.

• Drink a glass of fresh pineapple juice seasoned with a little salt each time, twice a day, to relieve thirst from fever.

Remarks: It is advisable to eat pineapple with a little salt to eliminate a slight itching at the tip of tongue.
• Bromelain in pineapple has been used to heal various types of inflammation, edema, and thrombus.
• Pineapple is not recommended for people with eczema or carbuncle.

Plum

Liver disease, diabetes, ascites.

Description: neutral; sweet and sour; produces fluids; promotes urination and digestion; affects the liver and kidneys.
Applications: Eat 2 fresh plums every day in the morning and evening to promote digestion and to arrest bleeding from gums.
• To cure cirrhosis and diminished urination, crush 2 sweet plums with seeds and mix with hot water. Drink like tea, 1 cup each time, twice a day.
• Soak fresh plums in vinegar to make vinegar plums.
• Crush 2 vinegar plums with their seeds, mix with boiling water and a little salt; let it cool down. Wash your mouth and throat with the juice a few times a day to cure chronic pharyngolaryngitis, tonsillitis, periodontitis, mouth canker, and tongue ulcer.
• Crush 30 g plum seeds and boil with water. Drink a cupful each time, twice a day, to relieve constipation.
Remarks: Plum is not recommended for people with weak stomachs, ulcers, and acute or chronic gastroenteritis.

Sour Plum

Diarrhea, dry cough, thirst.

Description: neutral; extremely sour; constrictive and obstructive; produces fluids and destroys worms; affects the liver.
Applications: Eat 2 fresh sour plums, or crush a fresh sour plum and mix with sugar and a little salt to make tea. Drink the tea to relieve thirst from fever and shortage of gastric acid and poor appetite.
• To make preserved sour plums (good for checking diarrhea), put ripe fresh sour plums in a large earthenware container; add salt, and marinate until the plums become so soft that juice begins to flow out.
Remarks: A friend who is now practicing acupuncture in Montreal told me that once he joined a group of people on an extreme diet and was told to eat a very large quantity of preserved plums every day. After a few days of consuming plums, he became so jumpy that while he was working at a store, he felt a strong urge to chase customers out and tell them to go to hell. The

plums can act upon the liver and thus, eating too many of them may disturb the liver and cause an emotional outbreak.

Apricot and Apricot Seed

Apricot for thirst and asthma; bitter apricot seed for cough, sore throat, constipation, asthma; sweet apricot seed for cough, constipation, and sore throat.

Description: Apricot is neutral, sweet and sour. Apricot lubricates the lungs and produces fluids. Bitter apricot seed is warm, pungent and bitter, and toxic. It is used to suppress cough, relieve asthma, and lubricate intestines. Sweet apricot seed is warm, pungent and sweet. It is used to lubricate the intestines and suppress a cough and also as an energy tonic.

Applications: Eat 2 to 3 fresh or dry apricots in the morning and evening to relieve a dry throat and to quench thirst.

• Chew 5 to 10 sweet apricot seeds once a day to cure chronic cough and shivering with cold.

• Combine 15 g sweet apricot seeds, 30 g each of rice and sugar; add water and crush them to make a cream. Eat it in the morning and evening to correct constipation in the elderly and in pregnant women.

• Prepare 2 pears and remove the seeds. Crush 6 g bitter apricot seeds and grind into powder; stuff the powder into the pears and steam for half an hour. Eat once a day to cure dry cough.

• Boil 9 g bitter apricot seeds in water with 6 g fresh ginger and 2 red dates. Drink as tea twice a day to cure a cough with watery mucus.

Remarks: Fresh apricots are not recommended for frequent or excessive consumption or for people with diarrhea. Bitter apricot seeds are toxic and should not be consumed in fresh or raw form.

Strawberry

Dry cough, thirst, sore throat, hoarseness, indigestion, difficulty when urinating, hangover.

Description: cool; sweet and sour; lubricates the lungs, produces fluids, strengthens spleen, relieves intoxication.

Applications: Steam 60 g fresh strawberries with 30 g rock sugar. Eat 3 times a day to treat dry cough which drags on and on.

• Drink a glass of fresh strawberry juice in the morning and evening, to relieve thirst in fever, sore throat, and hoarseness.

• Eat 60 g fresh strawberries before meals, 3 times a day, to relieve indigestion and abdominal pain and swelling, and to improve appetite.

• Crush 60 g fresh strawberries and mix with cold water. Drink a glass of the juice each time, 3 times a day, to relieve difficult and painful urination and discharge of red urine.
• Eat 8 to 10 fresh strawberries all at once to relieve hangover.
• Mix fresh strawberry juice with an equal amount of rice wine. Drink it to correct malnutrition and for weakness after illness.

Raspberry

Frequent urination, dizziness.

Description: warm; sweet and sour; used as a liver tonic and kidney tonic to control urination.
Applications: Drink fresh raspberry juice to stop frequent urination and dizziness due to motion sickness.
• Mix fresh raspberry juice with honey as a remedy to cure dry cough due to cold.
Remarks: Dry green (unripe) raspberry is an important Chinese herb with a neutral energy and sweet-sour flavor. It acts on the liver and kidneys, is used to correct impotence, seminal emission, frequent urination, blurred vision, and is reported to produce similar effects as those of a female sex hormone.

Date

Weak stomach, palpitations, nervousness, hysteria in women, allergic purpura.

Description: warm; sweet; used as a spleen tonic, energy tonic, and blood tonic; produces fluids; detoxicates; affects the spleen and stomach.
Applications: Boil 30 g red dates with 1 whole chicken egg, 4 fresh ginger slices, and 30 g brown sugar in water. Eat at meals to relieve weakness after childbirth.
• Prolonged consumption of 30 g red dates in the evening every day improves physical conditions, such as skinniness and weakness.
• Boil 30 g red dates with 5 green onion white heads. Eat it at bedtime to relieve insomnia.
• Eat 30 to 60 g red dates each time, 3 times a day for 15 consecutive days, to cure allergic purpura.
• Boil 30 g red dates and 30 g yam with 2 fresh ginger slices until soft. Eat it once a day for 10 consecutive days to treat cold stomachache, abdominal pain, and diarrhea due to digestive weakness.
• Boil 30 g dried red dates with 15 g yam, 15 g whole wheat, and 15 g processed

licorice. Drink the juice in the morning and evening to treat hysteria in women and jumpiness in women during menopause.
• Boil 15 g black dates with 9 g longans and 30 g brown sugar. Eat the stewed fruit at meals on a long-term basis to treat anemia.
• To prepare date jelly, boil 1,500 g fresh dates, seeded, or 500 g red dates, seeded, until they look like jelly; add 500 g sugar and stir until dissolved.
• Take a teaspoonful of date jelly with warm water on a long-term basis to relieve hepatitis, pulmonary tuberculosis, and weakness after illness.
Remarks: Fresh dates may be left in the sun to dry until red to make dried red dates.
• Fresh red dates may be boiled and left in the sun to dry, then steamed and baked a few times until the surface becomes quite black; these are called black dates.

Watermelon

Diminished urination, sore throat, mouth canker.

Description: cold; sweet; promotes urination and lubricates intestines; affects the heart, stomach, and bladder.
Applications: Drink a glass of fresh watermelon juice to relieve dizziness in sunstroke and vomiting.
• Eat 500 to 1,000 g fresh watermelon each time, twice a day, to relieve thirst, bitter taste in mouth, bad breath, discharge of yellowish urine, pain in urethra, and a hangover.
• Cut off watermelon peels about 0.5 cm thick and put them in the sun to dry, which become dry watermelon peels widely used as herb in Chinese herbalism.
• Boil 50 g of dry watermelon peels in water and drink as tea to treat hypertension, diabetes, nephritis, and a hangover.

Star Fruit (Carambola)

Cough and fever from a common cold, toothache, kidney and bladder stones, hemorrhoids, mouth canker, indigestion, hangover.

Description: cold; sweet and sour; reduces fever; produces fluids; promotes urination; detoxicates.
Applications: Eat a fresh star fruit each time, twice a day, to relieve fever and cough in common cold.
• Boil 3 fresh star fruits with 2 teaspoonfuls honey. Eat the fruits and drink the juice once a day to relieve kidney and bladder stones and difficult urination.

• Crush 3 fresh star fruits to make juice. Drink it twice a day to relieve pharyngolaryngitis, mouth canker, and toothache.
• Crush 3 fresh star fruits and mix the juice with cold water. Drink it 3 times a day to relieve painful urination and discharge of red urine.
• Eat 2 fresh star fruits each time, twice a day, first thing in the morning on an empty stomach and in the evening, to relieve hemorrhoids.

Longan

Insomnia, forgetfulness, palpitations, nervousness.

Description: warm; sweet; used as a spleen tonic, heart tonic, blood tonic, and energy tonic; affects the heart and spleen.
Applications: Steam 15 g longans with 30 g lean pork, 2 fresh ginger slices, and an adequate amount of rice wine. Eat once a day to relieve dizziness and underweight.
• Mix 500 g longans with 500 g sugar; steam them to make longan jelly.
• Take 1 spoonful longan jelly with warm water to relieve dizziness and edema after childbirth; or boil 15 g longans with 5 red dates, 30 g brown sugar, and 6 g fresh ginger. Drink it as soup once a day.

Lotus Fruit, Lotus Seed, and Lotus Root

Dreaminess, seminal emission, chronic diarrhea,
vaginal bleeding and discharge.

Description: neutral; sweet; obstructive; used as a spleen tonic, heart tonic, and kidney tonic; lotus root is also used as calmative; affects the heart, spleen, and kidneys.
Applications: Boil 30 g dried lotus fruits and 30 g brown sugar in 30 g rice wine; add 1 chicken egg as in egg-drop soup. Drink the soup every evening for 1 month to improve physical conditions after childbirth or excessive fatigue due to old age.
• Steam lotus fruits until cooked. Leave them in the sun to dry; grind into powder. Take 15 g of the powder each time, 3 times a day, to cure chronic diarrhea.
• Steam 250 g dried lotus fruits with 6 g rice wine and 6 g lard. Take the entire dosage 3 times a day for 1 month to cure ulcers or during the recovery stage after stomach bleeding.
• Mix 180 g lotus seeds and 30 g licorice and grind into powder. Take 3 to 6 g powder each time with warm water, 3 times a day, to relieve discharge of a short stream of red urine.
• Crush a few fresh lotus roots; squeeze out the juice. Drink a glass of the

juice each time to stop bleeding of various kinds, including nosebleed, vaginal bleeding, discharge of blood from anus, and vomiting of blood.

Remarks: It is interesting to note that lotus was referred to in Greek legend as yielding a fruit which induced a state of dreamy and contented forgetfulness in those who ate it. But in Chinese herbal remedies, it is believed that lotus fruit may be eaten to relieve dreaminess.

Lotus Plumule

Seminal emission, hypertension, blurred vision, swelling and pain in eyes.

Description: cold; bitter; obstructive; arrests bleeding; stops seminal emission; also used as a heart tonic; affects the heart, lungs, and kidneys.

Applications: Boil 3 g lotus plumule and drink it all at once to relieve seminal emission with or without dreams.

• Chew 1.5 g lotus plumule slowly and wash down with water to relieve hypertension.

• Boil 3 g lotus plumule and 3 g licorice with water. Drink it as tea, twice a day, to relieve anxiety and mouth canker.

Experiments: An experiment on animals shows that lotus plumule can lower blood pressure.

Remarks: Lotus plumule refers to the green bud of a ripe dry lotus seed.

Crab Apple

Diarrhea, diabetes, seminal emission.

Description: neutral; sweet and sour; quenches thirst; obstructive; affects the heart, liver, and lungs.

Applications: Boil 10 partially ripe fresh crab apples in an adequate amount of water until the water is reduced by half. Drink the soup and eat the crab apples first thing in the morning to cure watery diarrhea.

• Crush 60 g partially ripe fresh crab apples; boil crab apples in water. Drink a cup of the juice each time, 3 times a day, to relieve abdominal pain and diarrhea in enteritis and dysentery.

• Crush 15 to 30 g fresh crab apples; squeeze out the juice. Drink 3 times a day to cure diarrhea in children.

• Fry 30 g dried crab apples until yellowish; boil crab apples in water. Eat them at bedtime to cure seminal emission and premature ejaculation.

Remarks: It is not wise to consume crab apples in large quantities because they have an obstructive nature. Crab apples are not recommended for people with constipation.

Litchi (Lychee)

Hiccupping, stomachache, diarrhea, asthma, hernial pain.

Description: warm; sweet and sour; produces fluids; stimulates energy; relieves pain; affects the spleen and liver.

Applications: Eat 60 to 150 g fresh litchis to improve physical conditions after a prolonged illness.

• Fresh litchis may be left in the sun to dry. Dried litchis are widely used in the Chinese diet.

• Boil 30 to 60 g dried litchis and 5 dried red dates with adequate water. Drink the soup twice a day to cure chronic diarrhea.

• Steam 120 g dried litchis and eat once a day to cure asthma.

• Collect litchi seeds and leave them in the sun to dry to use in remedies.

• Crush 30 g dried litchi seeds; boil in water with 6 g fresh ginger or dried orange peels. Drink it once a day to relieve stomachache and abdominal pain.

• Crush 60 g dried litchi seeds and 15 g caraway seeds; boil them in an adequate amount of water. Drink the soup once a day to relieve hernial pain, elephantiasis, hydrocele of tunica vaginalis, and swelling and pain in the testes.

Walnut

Cough, lumbago, impotence, seminal emission, frequent urination, kidney and bladder stones, constipation.

Description: warm; sweet; used as kidney tonic and to lubricate intestines and check seminal emission; affects the kidneys and lungs.

Applications: Steam 30 g walnuts with 15 g rock sugar and 6 g radish seeds for half an hour. Eat the mixture twice a day to cure chronic asthma and cough.

• Chew 90 g of walnuts slowly each day to relieve sore throat, hoarseness, constipation, and gastric and duodenal ulcers.

• Boil 15 g walnut with 15 g crushed fresh ginger. Drink it twice a day to relieve headache and fever and fear of cold due to common cold, and also to induce perspiration in common cold.

• Steam 250 g walnuts and persimmon cakes each for 1 hour. Divide into 3 portions and eat 1 portion each time, 3 times a day, for 1 month to relieve cough and underweight due to pulmonary tuberculosis.

• Prepare 30 g walnuts, 2 pork kidneys, sliced, and a little lard; fry them together. Eat it hot every day at bedtime for 3 days to cure seminal emission with sudden urination.

• Fry 120 g walnuts in vegetable oil until crunchy. Mix walnuts with some sugar and water to make syrup. Eat it within 2 days to relieve stones in urinary tract.

Clinical report: For the treatment of kidney and bladder stones: Fry 120 g walnuts in vegetable oil until crunchy. Add sugar and grind into an emulsion or cream. Eat the walnuts within 1 to 2 days. (Reduce the dosage for children.) Treatment continues until stones are passed or the symptoms disappear. In general, stones are passed once or several times within a few days. They also appear smaller and softer than earlier stones or they are dissolved in urine to look like cream. Thus, walnut is considered effective for dissolving the stones.

Loquat

Pharyngolaryngitis, cough, thirst, constipation.

Description: cool; sweet and sour; lubricates the lungs; quenches thirst; pushes downwards; affects the spleen, lungs, and liver.

Applications: Steam 90 g fresh seeded loquats along with 15 g rock sugar for half an hour. Eat the loquats and drink soup to cure acute and chronic pharyngolaryngitis.

• Eat 250 g fully ripe loquats each time, in the morning and evening, to relieve dry throat and thirst and difficult urination.

• Crush 15 g loquat seeds; boil in water with 3 fresh ginger slices. Drink 1 cup of the juice each time, twice a day, to relieve coughing. Crush 9 to 15 g loquat seeds; boil seeds in water; strain and add 30 g honey and mix thoroughly. Drink once a day to cure senile constipation, cough, and asthma.

Remarks: Loquat is not recommended for people with weak digestions.

• Dried loquat leaf is an important Chinese herb with a cool energy and bitter flavor. It is used to relieve cough and nosebleed and coughing up blood.

Muskmelon

Cough, difficult urination, constipation, liver disease.

Description: cold; sweet; reduces fever; quenches thirst; promotes urination; affects the heart and stomach.

Applications: Eat 250 to 500 g muskmelon each time, twice a day, to relieve thirst in fever, pain on urination, and constipation.

• Steam 250 g fresh muskmelon with an adequate amount of rock sugar. Eat twice a day to relieve cough in pulmonary tuberculosis.

• To make dried calyx and receptacle of muskmelon, cut off calyx and receptacle of a muskmelon and leave them in the shade to dry. This is an important Chinese herb whose extracts are reported to have been made into tablets for hepatitis.

Remarks: Muskmelon and seeds are not recommended for people with diarrhea and edema. Dried calyx and receptacle of muskmelon are not recommended for people with heart disease.

Chestnut

Upset stomach, diarrhea, weak legs, vomiting of blood, nosebleed, discharge of stools containing blood.

Description: warm; sweet; used as a stomach tonic, spleen tonic, and kidney tonic; promotes blood circulation and arrests bleeding; affects the spleen, stomach, and kidneys.

Applications: Slowly chew 30 to 60 g fresh raw chestnuts (with shells removed) as chewing gum to cure chronic pharyngolaryngitis.
• Boil 30 to 60 g fresh or dried chestnuts in water with some brown sugar. Eat chestnuts at bedtime to relieve weakness and numbness of limbs.
• Bake 30 g dried chestnuts. Eat them in the morning and evening to cure frequent urination and weak legs due to kidney weakness.
• Boil 60 g fresh chestnuts with 4 red dates and some lean pork. Eat it all at once to cure asthma and cough.
• Crush 15 g chestnuts and mix with a persimmon cake to make jelly and then cook it. Eat it to cure diarrhea in children.
• Chestnut shells may be left to dry in the sun to use for remedies.
• Bake dried chestnut shells until they look like charcoal; grind them into powder. Take 6 g of the powder with 30 g honey to relieve hemorrhoids.

Peanut

Dry cough, upset stomach, beriberi, shortage of milk secretion after childbirth.

Description: neutral; sweet; lubricates the lungs; considered good for stomach-ache; affects the spleen and lungs.

Applications: Fry 3 cups roasted peanuts until aromatic; soak 1 cup rice (any kind except sweet [glutinous]) in water for at least 2 hours; drain and add the peanuts and boil together in water until they become soft to make peanut-rice congee soup. Drink the soup once a day to relieve beriberi and to promote milk secretion.
• Roast peanuts and eat them to stimulate the appetite, lubricate the intestines, and relieve a dry cough.
• Consume fresh peanuts to relieve a cough with mucous discharge.
• Boil 100 g fresh peanuts with an equal amount of small red beans and red dates. Drink as soup at meals to relieve beriberi.

• Boil 100 g peanuts with 1 pork foreleg. Eat at meals to promote milk secretion after childbirth.

• Boil 1 glass peanuts with 3 glasses water over low heat for 3 hours; add a little rock sugar, and drink it on an empty stomach to relieve beriberi.

• Consume fresh peanuts on a regular basis to relieve deafness.

Experiments: Initial experiments indicate peanuts arrest bleeding in hemophilia patients. Subsequent experiments show peanuts can arrest various kinds except severe bleeding. It is also found that fried or roasted peanuts are 20 times less effective than raw peanuts and the effects of the outer brown skins of the peanut are 50 times stronger than the peanut itself.

Clinical report: For the treatment of chronic tracheitis: Boil 70 g of the outer layers of peanuts in water for about 10 hours. Strain it to obtain 100 ml of the liquid; add sugar. Drink 50 ml each time, twice a day, for 10 days as a treatment program. Among the 407 cases of chronic tracheitis treated, 74 cases show significant results, 230 cases show improvements, 95 cases show no effects.

Remarks: The outer layers of peanuts should not be removed if possible when peanuts are used in a Chinese remedy, unless otherwise specified.

• Eating large quantities of peanuts is considered harmful to the digestive functions and to the skin.

• Peanut oil is neutral and sweet, and is used to lubricate the intestines. Use a cotton ball to apply peanut oil to the scrotum region to relieve itching and wet sensations, 5 or 6 times a day, without washing with hot water.

6

Vegetables, Roots, and Gourds

Chinese Cabbage

Constipation; thirst due to intoxication; ulcers.

Description: neutral; sweet; glossy; promotes urination; beneficial to the kidneys and brain after prolonged consumption; affects the stomach and large intestine.

Applications: Squeeze 1 to 2 fresh Chinese cabbages to obtain the juice; warm it. Drink the juice twice a day for 10 days to treat gastric and duodenal ulcers.

Remarks: It is reported that Chinese cabbage contains vitamin U, which is effective for the treatment of ulcers, reportedly better than artificial vitamin U.

• Although Chinese cabbage is listed among foods with neutral energy, it is commonly regarded as a cold food, useful for hot symptoms, such as inflammation or ailments of various kinds. These include eye infections, sore throat, chest pain, cough with yellowish mucous discharge, difficult urination, abdominal swelling, and constipation. The symptoms must be hot symptoms, if they are to be treated by Chinese cabbage.

• It is reported that fresh Chinese cabbage juice can also relieve gas poisoning.

Carrot

Chronic diarrhea; cough; indigestion; difficulty when urinating.

Description: neutral; sweet; pushes downwards; used as a diuretic and digestive; affects the lungs and spleen.

Applications: Regular consumption of fresh or cooked carrot prevents night blindness.

• Boil carrot and red dates in water to make soup to treat whooping cough in children.
• Carrot may be cooked with parsley and water chestnut for facilitating eruption in measles.
• Fresh carrot juice may be used for external application to heal burns.
• Boil 5 g carrot seeds in 2 glasses water over low heat until water is reduced to 1 glass. Drink the soup to promote urination for treatment of edema.
• Bake the peels of carrots until they appear burned. Eat the peels while hot to relieve frequent urination at night. Divide 1 carrot into 3 dosages and eat them 3 times a day.
• To use carrot as a blood tonic, cook it with spinach and lotus roots in soup; or, cook carrot with tomatoes, onion, and beef; or, cook carrot with pork liver.
• For sharpening the vision, cook carrot with chicken liver or duck liver.
Experiment: Shows the effect of lowering blood sugar in animals.
Remarks: I remember one day my friend told me that his 3-year-old son had wet the bed the previous night. I asked him casually if his son ate any carrot before going to bed. Quite unexpectedly, this friend was taken by surprise. "How did you know?" he asked. I told him that carrot can promote urination. In fact, carrot is also good to promote the outbreak of rash in measles, and for inflammation of the bladder and the kidneys not only because carrot is a diuretic, but also because it is an effective food for healing inflammations.

Celery

Hypertension, dizziness and headache, discharge of urine containing blood.

Description: neutral; sweet; bitter; glossy; affects the stomach and liver.
Applications: Sometimes an infant may feel hot sensations and is unable to sleep and cries day and night. If there are signs of hot symptoms (like mouth canker or redness in the region surrounding the anus or frequent urination with discharge of scanty and yellowish-red urine), then it is useful to cut a few pieces of celery, immerse them in boiling water for a few seconds and squeeze out the juice. This juice can reduce heat in the bladder, a useful remedy for urethritis.
• There is a Chinese recipe to improve the conditions of liver and kidneys: Fry celery and pork kidneys. The celery can calm you down and prevent liver disorder while the pork kidneys can tone up the kidneys.
• Celery is aromatic, the reason why the Chinese people call it "aromatic celery." Celery may be cooked with vinegar to lower blood pressure and relieve headache due to high blood pressure.
• Fresh celery juice may be mixed with honey to relieve dizziness and headache and shoulder pain associated with hypertension.

• In cases of hypertension of pregnancy and climacteric hypertension, drink fresh celery juice every day to relieve the symptoms.

Experiment: Celery lowers blood pressure in rats.

Clinical reports: A report on the effect of lowering blood pressure and the level of cholesterol: Wash fresh celery (with roots removed) in cold water. Squeeze out the juice and mix the juice with an equal quantity of honey or syrup. Drink 40 ml warm juice each time, 3 times a day. Among the 16 cases treated, 14 cases were effective and 2 cases had no effects. The results indicated effectiveness for primary hypertension, hypertension in pregnancy, and climacteric hypertension. In general, blood pressure begins to drop after 1 day of treatment with subjective sensations, improved sleeping conditions, and increased urination.

• A clinical report on the effects of celery roots: As a treatment program, 10 celery roots are washed, crushed, and boiled in water with 10 red dates for oral consumption twice a day for 15 to 20 days. Among the 21 cases treated for hypertension and coronary sclerosis heart disease with the cholesterol level over 200 mg percent, it was found that the level of cholesterol was reduced between 8 and 75 mg percent in 14 cases. It was also observed that fresh roots produce better results than dry ones and that dosages are flexible.

Remarks: According to Chinese theory, celery is effective for hypertension because it acts upon the liver; one type of hypertension is associated with the liver.

• A physician wrote to me about the fact that celery contains sodium, which is considered bad for hypertension. Nevertheless, I would think that the quantity of sodium contained in celery (25 mg in 1 stalk) is too small to cause any harm.

• A classic Chinese food belief: Celery can reduce internal heat in children and also internal heat in adults due to intoxication.

Bamboo Shoot

Measles, mucous discharge.

Description: cold; sweet; glossy.

Remarks: Bamboo shoot is a valuable ingredient in cooking meats because it has a cold energy. When it is cooked with meat, the bamboo shoot neutralizes the effects of the warm or hot energy in meat and, therefore, strikes a balance between the 2 ingredients. Like mushroom, bamboo shoot is widely used in the Chinese meat cookery.

• Many centuries ago, a celebrated Chinese poet was so fond of the combination, he wrote a poem emphasizing that meats and bamboo shoots are the 2 most appreciated ingredients at his dinner table.

• As Western people consume a large quantity of meat every day, it is wise to use bamboo shoots when cooking.

• Some people suffer from a skin disease that seems hidden beneath the skin, so to speak, because it won't go away nor will it erupt to the surface. When this happens, bamboo shoot can speed up the eruption, so that one can get it over with. This is also why bamboo shoot is good for measles before eruption of the rash.

• Bamboo leaves have a cold energy and light-sweet flavor. The leaves produce fluids, promote urination, are good for difficult urination with discharge of short streams of red urine.

Beetroot

Congested chest, poor energy circulation.

Description: neutral; sweet; promotes menstruation; promotes downwards movements.

Asparagus

Cough, mucous discharge, swelling, various kinds of skin eruptions, shortage of milk secretion after childbirth.

Description: slightly warm; bitter and slightly pungent; promotes urination.
Experiment: An animal experiment shows the effects of asparagus in promoting urination, lowering blood pressure, expanding terminal blood vessels, and reducing heartbeats.

Chive

Chest pain; difficulty when swallowing; upset stomach; vomiting blood; nosebleed; discharge of urine containing blood; prolapse of anus; injuries from a fall, causing internal blood coagulations.

Description: warm; pungent; promotes energy circulation; counteracts blood coagulations; affects the liver, stomach, and kidneys.
Contraindications: eye diseases and skin eruptions.
Applications: Squeeze the juice from fresh chive (leaves or roots). Drink 1 teaspoonful of the warm juice each time with milk to treat difficulty when swallowing. The same juice, cold without milk, is effective to treat sunstroke and also to wash skin eruptions caused by lacquer poisoning.

• Cook chive with pork or lamb liver to cure excessive perspiration and stimulate the appetite.

• Crush chive leaves or roots and externally apply the juice to the wound to relieve bruises, swelling, and pain.

• Cut chive leaves and roots into small pieces; boil with wine. Drink it hot to relieve injuries resulting from twisting the waist.

• Cook chive with egg to relieve diarrhea, night sweat, and nocturia.

Remarks: Chive is an important food for external injuries because it can counteract blood coagulations. When a person gets hurt (like in an automobile accident) he or she may feel pain long after the accident caused by internal blood coagulations not diagnosed by X-ray examination. The blood coagulation that is causing pain may be so light that it cannot be seen on the X ray. One useful way to determine whether blood coagulation occurred or not, however, is to determine if the pain recurs in the same body region or if it shifts around; if the patient always feels pain in the same region, it is very likely that blood coagulation has occurred, which may be relieved by eating chive. The Chinese people believe that pain may be caused either by blood coagulations or energy congestion. (When blood fails to circulate, it coagulates; when energy fails to circulate, it gets congested.) When pain is caused by blood coagulations, it will recur in the same region; when caused by energy congestion, the pain will shift around.

Here's a convenient way to use chive to relieve pain caused by blood coagulations: Cut chive into small pieces; boil it in water with wine and then drink the whole thing as soup. For example, in the past, Chinese authorities used to severely beat prisoners to force a confession from them but the severe beating caused internal bleeding and subsequently, internal blood coagulations. To prevent blood coagulations, it had become a routine practice to give prisoners chive at meals after the beating.

• Chive is warm in energy and acts upon the stomach. Therefore, chive is often used to relieve stomachache of a cold nature. As a matter of fact, the Chinese people always make a point of regularly eating chive, which is also effective for enteritis, if they have weak digestive functions. Fresh chive juice may also be drunk to relieve nosebleed (but its awful taste often makes the juice difficult to administer).

Chive Seed

Impotence, seminal emission with erotic dreams, frequent urination, uncontrolled or involuntary urination, diarrhea, vaginal discharge.

Description: warm; pungent and salty; affects the liver and kidneys.

Applications: For men having a strong erection with stinging pain in the penis, take 10 g chive seed ground into powder, with warm water each time, 3 times a day.

• For impotence and sexual weakness, boil over low heat 15 g chive seeds in 2 glasses water until reduced to 1 glass. Drink it as soup, 3 times a day; alternatively take about 20 chive seeds with salt water first thing in the morning (which should produce the same results).

Remarks: Chive seed is an important herb in Chinese herbal remedies and it is normally used as a yang tonic.

Chive Root

Chest pain; vomiting of blood; vaginal discharge; nosebleed; internal blood coagulations caused by injuries from a fall.

Description: warm; pungent; warms up the internal region; promotes energy circulation; counteracts blood coagulations.
Applications: Chive root may be applied the same as chive stem, except that the root is normally not used in cookery.

Chicory

Icterohepatitis.

Description: affects the liver and gall bladder.
Experiment: The entire plant was found to excite the central nervous system and increase heart actions in animals. The roots were found to increase appetite and improve digestive functions.

Corn Silk (Corn Style and Stigma)

Edema in nephritis, beriberi; icterohepatitis, hypertension, gallstones, diabetes; vomiting of blood; nosebleed; cholecystitis; sinusitis; mastitis.

Description: neutral; sweet; promotes urination; affects the liver and gall bladder.
Applications: Boil 40 g corn silk and 40 g banana peel in water. Drink the juice cold to relieve hypertension, nosebleed, and vomiting of blood.
● Boil corn silk with watermelon peel and small red beans in water. Drink it as soup for relief of chronic nephritis with edema and ascites.
Clinical reports: A report on the treatment of chronic nephritis: Place 50 g dry corn silk in 600 ml warm water; boil it over low heat for 20 to 30 minutes until reduced to about 300 to 400 ml soup; strain and drink the soup once a day; or divide it and drink it a few times a day. This remedy was used to treat 9 cases of chronic glomerular nephritis under observation for 10 months. The results indicate that among the 9 cases treated, 3 cases show complete recovery, 2 improvements, and 4 significant results. Corn silk promotes urination, improves kidney functions, heals or reduces edema, and eliminates or reduces urinary albumin, according to the report.
Experiments: Corn silk promotes urination, lowers blood sugar, is beneficial to the gall bladder and arrests bleeding, according to experiments on animals.

Applications: Boil 40 g corn silk and 40 g banana peel in water. Drink the juice cold to relieve hypertension, nosebleed, and vomiting of blood.
• Boil corn silk with watermelon peel and small red beans in water. Drink it as soup for relief of chronic nephritis with edema and ascites.

Corn (Maize)
Difficult urination, weak heart.

Description: neutral; sweet; used as a stomach tonic; promotes urination; affects the stomach and large intestine.
Remarks: One source indicates that a regular consumption of corn makes the heart stronger and increases sexual capacities, according to an experiment on swallows.
• Boil 15 g corn kernels in 3 glasses water over low heat until water is reduced to 1 glass, or until water becomes reddish brown. Drink half a glass of the soup each time, twice a day, to relieve kidney disease.
• Boil 30 g fresh corn leaves over low heat for 20 minutes. Drink the soup to relieve difficulty when urinating.

Eggplant
Discharge of blood from anus, dysentery with discharge of blood, discharge of urine containing blood.

Description: cool; sweet; affects the spleen, stomach, and large intestine.
Applications: Boil in water white eggplants and drink the soup with honey to relieve cough.
• Bake some peel from a fresh eggplant until it appears black as charcoal on the outside but inside intact; mix with honey. Put it in the mouth like chewing gum to cure stomatitis.
Clinical report: Eggplant contains vitamin P, which can prevent hardening of blood vessels and is useful in the treatment of arteriosclerosis, a report from China indicates. According to the statistics, the elderly Chinese are much less susceptible to apoplexy caused by cerebrovascular accident than their Western counterparts, attributed to the Chinese habit of eating eggplant. The same report points out two reasons for the elderly Chinese to consume more eggplants: Eggplants are much less expensive than other vegetables or meats; and eggplants can be cooked softer than other vegetables or meats, therefore easier for the elderly Chinese to eat (as most of them have lost most of their teeth). In addition, the Chinese people in general are fond of eggplants because of the taste.

Remarks: Eggplant is considered obstructive to some extent, which explains why it can heal various kinds of bleeding. Further, it has a cool energy that stops bleeding. Fresh eggplant can also relieve mushroom poisoning.

Cucumber

Sore throat, pink eyes, inflammation, burns.

Description: cool; sweet, detoxicates; promotes urination and quenches thirst; affects the spleen, stomach, and large intestine.

Applications: Squeeze the juice from the cucumber or the leaf. Apply externally to the affected region to relieve burns.

• When cucumber becomes old, it appears yellowish. Cucumber may then be boiled as soup to alleviate dry cough in autumn (when people are more likely to develop cough due to a dry climate). The Chinese people believe that the lungs are most susceptible to the external energy of dryness in autumn.

Remarks: Cucumber is effective to relieve common acne, because common acne is due to excessive heat in the lungs and stomach. Since cucumber has a cool energy and acts upon the stomach, fresh cucumber may be eaten to cure acne.

• The Chinese people preserve cucumber and eat it as a vegetable to cleanse the blood, clear up internal heat to cure hot diarrhea or hot skin conditions. Cut a cucumber lengthwise, remove and discard the seed portion, and put the cucumber in the sun to dry.

Black Fungus

Discharge of blood from anus, dysentery with discharge of blood, vaginal bleeding, hemorrhoids.

Description: neutral; sweet; arrests bleeding; cools the blood; affects the stomach and the large intestine.

Applications: Drink black fungus cooked with wine to relieve or prevent blood coagulations after external injuries or after childbirth.

• Cook black fungus as soup to relieve hemorrhoids.

• Boil black fungus in water and add brown sugar. Drink to relieve vaginal bleeding.

Remarks: It is reported that black fungus has been used as a contraceptive with results: Boil 450 g black fungus in water until very soft; mash it with brown sugar to make a syrup. Take the syrup with yellow rice wine, twice a day, for 3 to 7 days after childbirth.

White Fungus

Cough, discharge of mucus with blood, chronic constipation.

Description: neutral; sweet with a light taste; glossy; produces fluids and lubricates the lungs.

Remarks: White fungus is also called snow fungus. It is considered an important yin tonic, good for insomnia, lung disease, liver disease, and poor appetite. As white fungus is glossy, it is not recommended for those suffering from diarrhea or seminal emission.

• It is customary to cook white fungus with lean pork over low heat for as long as 3 hours; or boil white fungus in water with rock sugar. Some people prefer to boil white fungus in chicken soup, which makes it more delicious.

• White fungus should not be used to relieve cough due to common cold.

Lettuce

Diminished urination, discharge of bloody urine, shortage of milk secretion.

Description: cool; bitter and sweet; promotes urination and milk secretion; affects the stomach and large intestine.

Remarks: It is believed that excessive consumption of lettuce will cause dizziness and pain in the eyes.

Lettuce Seed

Swollen scrotum, hemorrhoids, shortage of milk secretion after childbirth.

Description: cold; bitter; promotes milk secretion and urination.

Applications: Grind 30 seeds into powder and dissolve in wine. Drink it for shortage of milk secretion after childbirth; or cook equal amounts of lettuce seeds and sweet rice and add a little licorice to eat at meals.

Onion

External applications for ulcers and trichomonas vaginitis.

Description: in folk medicine, onion is used as a diuretic and expectorant.

Applications: Boil 10 g onion over low heat. Eat it to lower blood pressure.

• Eat onion regularly to increase muscular strength.

Experiments: Sauté 60 g onion with vegetable oil. Healthy males who eat the onion inhibit a rise in cholesterol caused by a high level of fat intake. Onion also acts to reduce fibrinolysis activity and is considered beneficial in the treatment of arteriosclerosis.

• An experiment on animals indicates that onion increases intestinal tension and secretion and is considered beneficial to weak intestines and nondysenteric enteritis.

Green Onion White Head

Headache, abdominal pain, constipation, suppression
of urination, dysentery.

Description: warm; pungent; induces perspiration; affects the lungs and stomach.

Applications: For relief of nasal congestion and nasal discharge in infants associated with common colds, steam a green onion white head and a mushroom with 30 to 50 ml mother's milk. Feed infants the soup without the mushroom or white head.

• Crush 4 to 6 white heads; warm it up with wine. Drink the soup to remedy a common cold.

Remarks: Green onion white head is an important herb in Chinese medicine. It can induce perspiration and warm the body. It is most frequently used to relieve common cold at its early stages.

Green Onion Leaf

Headache and nasal congestion associated with common cold.

Description: warm; pungent; induces perspiration.

Leek

Diarrhea in enteritis of large intestine, bleeding, dysphagia,
upset stomach.

Description: warm; pungent; obstructive; affects the liver and lungs.

Potato

Lack of energy, mumps, burns.

Description: neutral; sweet; heals inflammations; used as an energy tonic and a spleen tonic.

Applications: Crush a potato and squeeze out the juice; mix it with vinegar. Apply the juice to the affected region to relieve mumps.

• Apply potato juice externally to burns.

• Prepare 5 potatoes (the size of eggs), 1 onion, and an adequate amount of garlic and carrots. Wash and thoroughly clean the potatoes but do not peel them. Cut up the potatoes and onion; put all ingredients in about a few cups water; simmer over low heat until the water is reduced to half and add some salt. Drink 2 cups of the soup at each meal; or adjust the quantity and frequency according to individual needs. This soup is good for hypertension, malnutrition in infants, diarrhea, bronchial asthma, allergic skin, kidney disease, and also for obesity.

• To relieve gastric and duodenal ulcers, eat a cupful of cooked potato liquid with a spoon once a day. To make the potato remedy, wash 30 fresh unpeeled potatoes and grate them to squeeze out the juice. Simmer the juice in an earthenware pot (not a metal one) over low heat without a cover until the water evaporates completely to form a thick layer at the bottom of the pot. This substance is called potato glue and is full of protein. By taking this sticky liquid you can relieve pain and heal a sensitive stomach. It is reported that gastric and duodenal ulcers may recover within 20 to 30 days by taking this glue.

Sweet Potato

Stomach weakness, kidney weakness, premature ejaculation.

Description: neutral; sweet; used as a spleen and an energy tonic, and as a yin kidney tonic.

Applications: Apply sweet potato soup to the affected region to heal frostbite; or apply the steam of the boiling sweet potato by holding to the frostbitten region over the steam.

• Bake sweet potato until the surface is charred; grind into powder. Take 10 g of the powder dissolved in warm water to relieve common cold. Charred sweet potato can induce perspiration and reduce fever.

Remarks: When a child accidentally swallows a coin, feed the child large quantities of boiled sweet potatoes all at once; the coin will be coated by the sweet potatoes to discharge along with the stool.

Pumpkin

Bronchial asthma, cough, edema.

Description: neutral; sweet and slightly bitter.

Clinical report: More than 30 sufferers of bronchial asthma were given each day about a pound of steamed pumpkin mixed with honey and sugar. The majority of patients were able to control the symptoms with either an absence of asthma attacks or significant improvements. Some patients did not have recurring attacks during the observation periods, ranging from 6 months to

2 years. Preliminary observations indicated that the patients of simple bronchial asthma have the best results and patients of complicated bronchial asthma also show some improvements.

Radish

Abdominal swelling due to indigestion, laryngitis due to continual cough with mucous discharge, vomiting of blood, nosebleed, dysentery, headache.

Description: cool; pungent and sweet; affects the lungs and stomach; detoxicates; downwards movements; promotes digestion and eliminates hot mucous discharge.
Applications: Drink fresh radish juice mixed with ginger juice to cure laryngitis.
• Drink fresh radish juice to relieve intoxication.
• Regular consumption of fresh radishes prevents common cold, flu, and respiratory infections.

Radish Leaf

Chest congestion, hiccupping, indigestion, diarrhea, sore throat, swelling of breast in women, shortage of milk secretion.

Description: neutral; pungent and bitter; promotes digestion and energy circulation; affects the spleen and stomach.
Application: Cut up dry radish leaves, boil them in water and add some salt. Use the warm liquid to wash the genital areas in women to relieve itching, or pour the liquid into the bathtub and sit in it to relieve cold sensations in the genital region.

Taro Leaf

Diarrhea, excessive perspiration, night sweat.

Description: cool; pungent; checks perspiration and diarrhea; heals swelling.

Taro Flower

Stomachache, vomiting of blood, prolapse of uterus, hemorrhoids, prolapse of anus.

Description: neutral; numbing taste.
Remarks: Boil fresh taro flower in small quantities.

Taro

Tuberculosis of the lymph nodes, scrofula, external application to relieve inflammation, swelling, and pain.

Description: neutral; sweet and pungent; glossy; affects the stomach and large intestine.
Applications: Peel about 30 fresh taros (roots); cut into pieces and fry in vegetable oil. Dry taro in the sun; grind into powder. Take 15 g of the powder dissolved in warm water each time, twice a day, to cure scrofula.

Tomato

Thirst, poor appetite, hypertension, constipation.

Description: slightly cold; sweet and sour; produces fluids; promotes digestion.
Applications: Eat 1 or 2 fresh tomatoes first thing in the morning on an empty stomach to relieve hypertension and bloodshot eyes.
• Boil tomato juice with ginger juice and drink it as soup to prevent blood coagulations after injuries.
• Cook 2 tomatoes with 60 g pork liver to relieve night blindness.
• Eat 1 fresh tomato sweetened with sugar twice a day to relieve bleeding gums.
• Eat 1 or 2 fresh tomatoes twice a day; or cook tomatoes with pork and eat it to quench thirst and improve appetite.

Lily Flower

Insomnia, cough, nervousness.

Description: cool; sweet; lubricates the lungs; relieves nervousness; affects the lungs.
Applications: Boil 40 g lily flowers for half an hour and sweeten with sugar. Drink the juice at bedtime to cure insomnia.
Remarks: Lily flower is referred to by the Chinese people as the "sorrow-forgetting flower" because it can relieve nervousness and let you forget your sorrow.

Bitter Gourd (Wild Cucumber)

Sunstroke, dysentery, pink eyes and pain in eyes.

Description: cold; bitter; detoxicates; sharpens the vision; affects the heart, spleen, and stomach.

Applications: Fry bitter gourd seeds and grind into powder. Take 10 g of the powder dissolved in wine each time, twice a day, to cure impotence.
• Regular consumption of bitter gourd improves eyesight.
Remarks: Bitter gourd is regarded as the king of bitter foods. It is bad for people with a weak stomach because it could cause vomiting. But it is good for those with a hot physical constitution as it can cool down the internal region and relieve hot constipation.
• According to Chinese medical theory, bitter foods can improve the conditions of the liver (which is why bitter gourd is good for liver disease).

Spinach

Nosebleed, discharge of blood from anus, thirst in diabetes, constipation, alcoholism, scurvy, hemorrhoids.

Description: cool; sweet; glossy; lubricates dryness, arrests bleeding, used as a blood tonic; affects the large and small intestines.
Application: Immerse spinach in boiling water for 3 minutes and eat it with a little sesame oil to treat hypertension, constipation, headache, and dizziness.
• Simmer large quantities of spinach, including roots and heads, over low heat for 2 or 3 hours. Drink it as tea to relieve a hangover and alcoholism.
Remarks: Spinach is not recommended for persons with premature ejaculation and diarrhea because it is glossy (sliding). But it is good for skin eruptions caused by a hot physical constitution.
• Spinach can cleanse the blood and is good for many hot skin eruptions and itchy skin, which are caused by hot blood in many instances. Spinach also has a cool energy. To treat hot skin diseases, spinach may be cooked with seaweed or kelp, which also can cleanse the blood.
• In summer when the weather is really hot, if some people develop sore throat or chest congestion after eating fried foods, it is beneficial to drink some spinach soup.

Shiitake Mushroom

Prevention of rickets, anemia, measles.

Description: neutral; sweet; affects the stomach.
Applications: Boil some shiitake mushrooms in water until the soup becomes yellowish. Drink only the liquid (without eating the mushrooms) to relieve vomiting caused by careless eating; another alternative is to place shiitake mushrooms in boiling water and steep until the soup becomes yellowish. Drink it as tea.

• Dissolve some sugar or honey in the shittake mushroom soup to treat coughing.

• Drink shiitake mushroom soup, or dissolve shiitake mushroom powder in hot water and drink it as tea to relieve fish poisoning. A prolonged consumption by this method is believed to prevent arteriosclerosis.

• In case of difficult urination or discharge of urine containing blood, bake some shiitake mushroom until it appears burned on the surface. Eat 10 g each time, twice a day, or eat fresh shiitake mushrooms.

Experiment: Studies with rats show shiitake mushroom lowers blood fat levels.

Clinical report: Shiitake mushroom counteracts cholesterol, a recent report indicates.

Remarks: Shiitake mushroom is believed to counteract stomach and cervical cancers. (When I visited Japan in October 1985, I learned that a new product containing the extract from shiitake mushroom had been approved by the Japanese government as an anti-cancerous agent.) The Chinese people are very fond of mushrooms, including shiitake mushrooms, which are produced primarily in Japan. Shiitake mushroom may be cooked by itself and it may also be cooked with other vegetables. In either case, avoid excessive amounts of soy sauce and salt because they are quickly absorbed by the mushroom and spoil its good taste.

Button Mushroom

Diarrhea, mucous discharge, vomiting.

Description: cool; sweet; affects the stomach, lungs, and intestines.

Applications: Cook common button mushroom to relieve leukocytopenia and contagious hepatitis and to prevent metastasis after a cancer operation.

Experiment: Common button mushroom has the effects of antibiosis and lowers blood fat, according to an experiment.

Wax Gourd (Winter Gourd or Winter Melon)

Edema, beriberi, sunstroke, hemorrhoids, alcoholism.

Description: cool; sweet and light tastes; detoxicates; promotes urination; eliminates mucus; affects the lungs, bladder, and small and large intestines.

Applications: Drink fresh wax gourd juice to relieve sunstroke and thirst.

• Cook 100 g dry wax gourd peel until it becomes syrup. Drink it in large quantities each day to relieve all kinds of edema associated with diminished urination, including kidney disease, heart disease, beriberi, and cirrhotic ascites.

• Boil 100 g wax gourd over low heat. Drink it as soup. Or bake a wax gourd until its skin appears charred. Take 30 g each time, twice a day. Or eat cooked wax gourd on a regular basis to promote urination and bowel movements, cure edema, beriberi, and hemorrhoids.

Remarks: Chinese wax gourd peel is commonly used in Chinese medicine. It may be used as wax gourd but with greater effects.

Squash

Pulmonary abscess, bronchiectasis, roundworms, opium addiction.

Description: warm; sweet; heals inflammation; relieves pain; affects the spleen and stomach.

Applications: Drink fresh squash juice frequently to relieve opium addiction.

• Cook 400 g squash with 200 g beef without salt or oil. Eat it to cure pulmonary abscess and bronchiectasis.

• Apply fresh squash juice to burns.

Clinical report: Consumption of 400 g fresh squash (reduced by half in children) followed by taking a purgative 2 hours later, once a day for 2 consecutive days, was found to expel roundworms (from 2 to over 100) in 6 out of 10 cases.

• Squash seeds have been found to expel tape worms, roundworms, and blood flukes.

• Prepare 20 g squash seeds and remove the shells; wrap the seeds in a cloth and crush them. Mix it with water or with a little soy sauce or sugar. Drink it in the morning and evening for 3 to 5 days. This has been found to promote milk secretion after childbirth; but fully cooked seeds have not been found effective.

• Squash leaves are effective for dysentery. Boil 10 leaves with a little salt. Drink it as tea twice a day to relieve dysentery.

• Squash flowers may be boiled to drink as tea to cure jaundice and cough.

Remarks: Squash is not recommended for people suffering from chest congestion or water retention.

Kohlrabi

Indigestion, jaundice, diabetes, alcoholism, nosebleed.

Description: neutral; bitter, sweet and pungent; detoxicates.

Applications: Drink fresh kohlrabi juice to stop nosebleed.

• Crush fresh kohlrabi seeds into powder. Take 10 g powder each time, twice a day, to relieve difficult urination after childbirth and improve the eyesight.

• Crush 10 g kohlrabi seeds into powder. Mix with a glass of boiling water. Strain through cheesecloth over a bowl and squeeze out all the liquid. Drink the liquid as tea first thing in the morning to induce bowel movements and urination.

Leaf Mustard

Mucous discharge, cough, chest congestion.

Description: warm; pungent; affects the lungs.

Applications: Cook preserved leaf mustard and eat 30 g a day to cure pulmonary abscess and bronchiectasis and laryngitis. Boil 5 g fried leaf mustard seeds with 10 g fried radish seeds, 5 g dried orange peel and 5 g licorice. Drink it as tea to cure chronic bronchitis and cough with mucous discharge.

Remarks: A prolonged consumption of leaf mustard can warm up the internal region. It is not recommended for people suffering from eye diseases, hemorrhoids, or discharge of stools containing blood, which are normally regarded as hot symptoms.

• Leaf mustard can relieve congestion because it has a warm energy and tastes pungent, which are the two important components of foods that are used to promote energy circulation and relieve congestion of various kinds.

Yam

Chronic diarrhea, cough, diabetes, seminal emission,
vaginal discharge, frequent urination.

Description: neutral; sweet, spleen tonic, lung tonic, and kidney tonic; affects the lungs, spleen, and kidneys.

Applications: Prepare 80 g raw yam and grind into powder. Wash an equal amount of glutinous (sweet) rice and drain it; put rice in the sun to dry. Toast the rice in a pan, shaking or stirring, until yellowish and grind into powder. Mix the yam and rice. Take 4 spoonfuls of the powder, some sugar, and black pepper dissolved in warm water each morning to treat chronic diarrhea and poor appetite.

• Boil yam with ginseng for 30 minutes and drink it as tea. Or make a soup with yam and beef or pork.

Water Chestnut

Diabetes, jaundice, urinary strains, pink eyes,
sore throat, hypertension.

Description: cold; sweet; relieves fever and indigestion; promotes urination; affects the lungs and stomach.

Applications: Boil 5 water chestnuts in water with 1 fresh mandarin orange peel. Drink as tea, 3 times a day, to relieve hypertension.

• Peel 100 g water chestnuts and chew them slowly in the morning and evening; or drink water chestnut juice to cure sore throat, hemorrhoids, and mouth canker.

• Prepare 500 g water chestnuts; wash in water and dry thoroughly; put them in half a bottle of rice wine; seal it and set aside for a few days. Slowly chew 2 water chestnuts each time and wash down with the rice wine in the bottle, twice a day, to cure diarrhea with discharge of whitish or reddish substances.

• Warm a glass of water chestnut juice and mix with 2 teaspoonfuls rice wine. Drink it to relieve discharge of blood from anus (as in hemorrhoids).

7
Legumes, Grains, Oils, and Seeds

Barley

Indigestion, diarrhea, pain when urinating, edema, burns.

Description: cool; sweet and salty; regulates the stomach; expands the intestines; promotes urination; affects the spleen and stomach.

Applications: Fry barley until aromatic and slightly brown. Use it to make tea to relieve summer heat, indigestion, fatigue, and excessive perspiration in summer.

• Fry 1 cup barley until aromatic and slightly brown to make tea with a few slices of fresh ginger. Drink it as a substitute for regular tea or juice, which is good for people who feel thirsty in hot weather but cannot drink tea or juice for one reason or another.

• Boil 100 g barley in water and mix with fresh ginger juice to drink before meals to cure difficult urination and pain when urinating.

• Fry barley until charred; grind into powder and mix in vegetable oil for external application to relieve burns.

• Regular consumption of barley cures uremia and indigestion.

• Boil 5 g tender barley leaves and stalks. Drink as tea to promote urination.

Malt

Indigestion, abdominal swelling, poor appetite, vomiting, diarrhea, swelling of breasts.

Description: slightly warm; sweet; promotes digestion; pushes downwards; affects the spleen and stomach.

Applications: Boil 50 g malt in water and drink as soup to cure indigestion, abdominal swelling, and swelling of breast with pain.

• Boil 50 g malt with 10 g orange peel in water. Drink as tea to relieve the aftereffects of acute and chronic hepatitis.

• Fry malt and grind into powder. Take 2 teaspoonfuls with wine each time, twice a day, to cure abdominal swelling and tightness after childbirth; or take 2 teaspoonfuls with warm water each time, twice a day, to relieve fever after childbirth or shortage of milk after childbirth, or swelling of breasts after childbirth.

• Boil 40 g each of fresh malt and fried malt. Drink as soup once a day for three consecutive days to cure swelling of breasts at weaning; if swelling and hardness and pain are observed, double the quantities of fresh malt and fried malt.

• Boil 10 g hawthorn fruits and 10 g fried malt (to be reduced in case of children), and drink as tea, 3 times a day, to relieve indigestion.

Clinical report: For treatment of acute and chronic hepatitis: Prepare tender roots of malt sprouts. (To make malt sprouts, wash barley, then immerse in water for 12 hours; drain, then wrap tightly in a wet cloth and splash water on them a few times daily until they sprout; dry the sprouts in the sun.) Dry and grind into powder and mix with syrup for a remedy. Take 10 ml (containing 15 g malt powder) each time, 3 times a day, after meals; in addition, an adequate amount of yeast and vitamin B-complex tablets should be administered. In general, one treatment program consists of 30 days, and one additional treatment program should be administered after recovery. Among the 161 cases treated, 108 cases showed effects and 53 cases showed no effects, which means the effective rate is 67.1 percent. Among the subjects treated, of the 56 cases of acute hepatitis, 48 cases showed effects of the treatment; of the 105 cases of chronic hepatitis, 60 cases showed effects. After treatments, there are decreases of various degrees in symptoms, such as pain in liver, anorexia, fatigue, and low temperature, particularly the symptom of anorexia. Among the cases that showed effects, there are various degrees of decreases in the size of a swollen liver and in transaminase. A few patients showed some side effects, including dry sensations in the mouth, bitter taste in the mouth, anxiety, and diarrhea. The long-term effects of this treatment should be determined by further research.

Maltose

Fatigue, abdominal pain, dry cough, thirst, vomiting of blood, sore throat, constipation.

Description: warm; sweet; slows down the attack of acute symptoms; produces fluids; lubricates dryness; also used as an energy tonic; affects the spleen, stomach, and lungs.

Applications: Take a few teaspoonfuls of maltose with warm water several

times a day to neutralize the effects of drug overdose and to relieve pain from chronic gastric and duodenal ulcers and stomachache.
• Shape maltose into a ball as large as an egg yolk and swallow it to dislodge a fishbone stuck in the throat; a few balls may be necessary and the ball of maltose gradually may be increased in size each time.
• Bake maltose until partially browned. Take 1 teaspoonful dissolved in warm water each time, twice a day, to relieve a sore throat; or, mix maltose with crushed carrot; marinate overnight; next day, mix with water and drink 1 glass each time, 3 times a day.

Hyacinth Bean

Diarrhea and vomiting in summer, vaginal discharge, malnutrition in children.

Description: neutral; sweet; used as a spleen tonic; reduces water retention; affects the spleen and stomach.
Applications: Grind hyacinth beans into powder. Take 15 g of the powder dissolved in warm water each time, 3 times a day, to cure acute gastroenteritis, vomiting, and diarrhea; or boil 50 g hyacinth beans and drink as soup, 3 times a day. The same remedy may also be used to cure difficulty when urinating.
• Grind hyacinth beans into powder. Take 15 g of the powder dissolved in rice soup each time, 3 times a day, to relieve quickening in women due to taking drugs; or, drink concentrated juice of hyacinth bean, twice a day.
• Cook a bowl of hyacinth beans with sugar, and eat it at meals to cure chronic diarrhea.

Broad Bean (Horse Bean)

Edema, tinea capitis.

Description: neutral; sweet; used as a spleen tonic; eliminates water retention; affects the spleen and stomach.
Applications: Boil 70 g broad beans and 70 g wax gourd peels in water. Drink as tea to cure edema.
• Crush fresh broad beans into a cream. Apply externally to the affected region to relieve tinea capitis; or use dried broad beans, if necessary.
• Dry fresh broad beans in the sun to grind into powder. Take 2 teaspoonfuls of the powder dissolved in warm water each time, 3 times a day, to cure diarrhea and discharge of stools containing blood.
• Boil broad bean powder with sugar in water. Drink as tea to relieve poor appetite and diarrhea in children (white sugar should be used in the absence

of discharge of blood but brown sugar in the presence of blood from the anus). The older the powder is, the better its effects will be.

Castor Bean

Carbuncle, swelling, tuberculosis of the lymph node, sore throat, edema, constipation.

Description: neutral; sweet and pungent; heals swelling with its detoxicating effects; induces bowel movements; affects the large intestine and lungs.
Applications: Grind 20 uncooked castor beans (shells removed) and add a little salt to apply to cure swelling of a carbuncle.
• Fry castor beans in vegetable oil until fully cooked; peel the beans. Chew 3 beans at bedtime and gradually increase to 10 or more beans each time, to relieve tuberculosis of the lymph node.
Clinical report: For treatment of facial paralysis: Grind castor beans (shells removed) to make into a cream. Apply externally to the affected side of the mandibular joint and angle of mouth (the layer of cream should be 3-mm or about ⅛-in. thick) and covered with a bandage; change dressing once every day. Among the 3 cases treated, all recovered within 3 days.
• A report on castor bean poisoning and treatment: The toxic substances in castor beans are destroyed by heat. Most cases of castor bean poisoning are due to consumption of fresh castor beans. A report indicates that 3 children who ate 2 to 7 fresh castor beans vomited continually, with abdominal pain; one child suffered from unclear consciousness with dehydration, cold limbs, enlargement of the pupils, and poor reactions to light. All cases recovered after treatment by standard procedures of treating poisoning.
Remarks: Castor bean oil (castor oil) is good for constipation but bad for the stomach. For that reason, pregnant women should avoid castor oil.

Small Red Bean (Adzuki Bean)

Edema, beriberi, jaundice, diarrhea, discharge of blood from anus, carbuncle swelling, mumps, cirrhotic ascites.

Description: neutral; sweet and sour; facilitates urination; heals swelling; detoxicates; affects the heart and small intestine.
Applications: Boil 100 g small red beans in water with 300 g wax gourd. Drink as soup at meals once a day to relieve nephritis, beriberi, and trophedema.
• Grind small red beans into powder and mix with honey. Apply to a carbuncle to heal the swelling.

• Boil 100 g small red beans in water. Eat at meals to promote milk secretion after childbirth.
• Fry 300 g small red beans until charred. Add 6 bowlfuls of water and boil until water is reduced to 3 bowlfuls. Add some brown sugar as seasoning. Drink 1 bowl of soup each time, 3 times a day, to relieve abdominal pain due to blood coagulations after childbirth.

Clinical report: For a treatment of cirrhotic ascites: Boil 1 pound of small red beans with a common carp (more than 1 pound) in 2 to 3 L water until the beans break. Eat the beans and fish, and drink the soup separately, daily or every other day until cured. Results of 2 cases treated showed increased urination and reduced abdominal size, with good spirits and no side effects.
• A report on the treatment of mumps: Grind 50 to 70 small red beans into powder; mix it with warm water and egg white or honey to make a cream to apply to the affected region; cover it with a bandage. In general, swelling disappears with one treatment; all 7 cases treated showed good results.

Remarks: There are many kinds of ordinary red beans that should be distinguished from small red beans under discussion. Ordinary red beans are round in shape whereas small red beans are long. Ordinary red beans have a neutral energy, bitter flavor, are normally used to promote energy circulation and menstrual flow, and are considered good for hernia, abdominal pain, and the suppression of menstruation.

Kidney Bean

Edema, beriberi.

Description: neutral; sweet and light taste; promotes urination; heals swelling.
Application: Boil 150 g kidney beans with 15 g garlic and 40 g sugar in water. Drink as soup at meals to relieve edema.

Sword Bean

Hiccupping, vomiting, abdominal swelling, lumbago due to kidney deficiency, mucous discharge.

Description: warm; sweet; pushes downwards; warms the internal region; used as a kidney tonic; affects the stomach and large intestine.
Applications: Boil 30 g old dried sword beans with shell, along with 3 slices fresh ginger; strain it to obtain juice, and add some brown sugar. Drink 1 cup each time, 3 times a day, to relieve hiccupping and coughing.
• Cook 50 g sword beans with a pork kidney. Eat them at meals once every

other day to relieve lumbago due to weak kidneys and during pregnancy.
• Fry sword beans until browned; grind into powder. Take 4 g powder each time with rice wine, 3 times a day, to cure headache, intercostal neuralgia, and pain caused by injuries.
• Boil 20 g sword beans in water; strain and add rock sugar or honey. Drink it as tea once a day to relieve whooping cough in children and asthma and cough in the elderly.

String Bean (Green Bean)

Diarrhea, vomiting, diabetes, seminal emission, whitish vaginal discharge, frequent urination.

Description: neutral; sweet; used as a kidney tonic and a spleen tonic; affects the spleen and kidneys.
Application: Boil 50 g dried string beans (with the shells) in water. Drink as soup once a day to relieve diabetes, thirst, and frequent urination.

Mung Bean

Edema, diarrhea, drug poisoning, erysipelas.

Description: cool; sweet; detoxicates; reduces hot sensations of the body; promotes urination; affects the heart and stomach.
Applications: Boil 200 g mung beans in water; add a little honey or sugar as a seasoning. Drink as soup at meals, once a day, to cure red skin eruptions and urination difficulty due to fever; or grind mung beans into powder and take 15 g powder dissolved in warm water each time, twice a day.
Clinical reports: A treatment of pesticide poisoning: Crush 500 g mung beans and mix with 60 g salt in about 2 L cold water for a few minutes; strain and drink as much as possible, but no more than 3 to 5 L each day. The 15 cases treated all recovered within 24 hours. No side effects were observed with the exception of occasional vomiting.
• A report on the treatment of lead poisoning: Boil 15 g mung beans with 16 g licorice to eat twice daily with 300 mg vitamin C added each time. Each treatment program lasts 10 to 15 days. A total of 9 cases of light poisoning and 28 cases of lead absorption were treated and all the cases showed basic recovery.
Remarks: Mung bean sprouts have a cold energy and sweet flavor and are used to counteract alcoholism and heat in the body.
• Mung bean powder may be used for the same purpose as mung bean. Its particular uses are for burns, alcoholism, and food poisoning.

Rice Bran

Difficulty when swallowing, beriberi.

Description: neutral; sweet and pungent; pushes downwards; affects the stomach and large intestine.

Applications: Mix rice bran with honey and shape into tablets. Keep 1 tablet at a time in the mouth just as a cough drop. This remedy relieves difficulty when swallowing.

• Fry 250 g rice bran until yellowish but not burned. Store in a jar for application. Take 10 g of the yellowish rice bran with water each time, twice a day, to relieve beriberi.

Polished (White) Rice

Diarrhea, morning sickness, difficult urination.

Description: neutral; sweet; used as an energy tonic and a spleen tonic; affects the spleen and stomach.

Applications: Fry 1 bowlful polished rice with fresh ginger juice until the rice becomes yellowish. Chew 20 to 30 grains before getting up in the morning to relieve morning sickness.

• Boil rice in water as you would normally, but cook it a little longer than usual to allow a thick crust of charred rice to form on the bottom of the pan; rice is neutral, and bitter and sweet.

• Boil 150 g browned crust of rice with an equal amount of lotus fruits and sugar in an adequate amount of water. Drink 2 teaspoonfuls each time, 3 times a day, to cure diarrhea, particularly in children.

Sweet (Glutinous) Rice

Excessive urination, excessive perspiration, diarrhea.

Description: warm; sweet; used as an energy tonic; affects the spleen, stomach, and lungs.

Applications: Fry sweet rice with wheat bran and grind into powder. Take 10 g powder in warm water each time, 3 times a day, to stop excessive perspiration.

• Cook 50 g sweet rice with 60 g Job's tears and 8 red dates. Eat at meals to relieve pulmonary tuberculosis, neurasthenia, anemia, and various kinds of chronic diseases.

• Boil sweet rice sprouts in water with malt. Drink the soup to relieve indigestion and to promote appetite.

Bean Curd (Tofu)

Pink eyes, diabetes, periodic diarrhea, sulfur poisoning.

Description: cool; sweet; used as an energy tonic; produces fluids; lubricates dryness; detoxicates; affects the spleen, stomach, and large intestine.

Applications: Prepare 1 bowl bean curd, 70 g maltose, and half a cup of fresh radish juice; combine the 3 ingredients in a pan, add half a cup of water, and bring to a boil once. Divide the soup into 2 dosages and drink twice a day to treat asthma with mucous discharge, including acute bronchial asthma.

• Crush a number of bean curds and apply the mash to the legs to heal erysipelas on the legs; change the dressing as soon as the mash dries.

Yellow Soybean

Malnutrition in children, diarrhea, abdominal swelling, underweight, gestosis.

Description: neutral, sweet; used as a spleen tonic; lubricates dryness; eliminates tissue fluids; affects the spleen and large intestine.

Applications: Fry yellow soybeans until aromatic to eat at meals to promote milk secretion after childbirth.

• Fry yellow soybeans and then boil them in water to eat at meals to correct underweight.

Clinical report: A treatment of acute gestosis: 92 cases of potential eclampsia and eclampsia are treated by soybean juice (soybean and water ratio 1 to 8) cooked with 120 g sugar, divided into 6 dosages. Eat while drinking additional water. In general, treatment lasts 2 to 4 days, and then, changes to a salt-free diet. On the second day of treatment, fruits or lotus root powder may be administered to relieve hunger. In the control group, 41 cases are given only a salt-free diet with other factors identical in both groups, including avoidance of sound and light stimuli, and administration of sedatives and antispasmodic drugs. The results indicate that the experimental group shows a faster disappearance of edema and faster normalization of the blood pressure than the control group; the death rate in the experimental group is zero while in the control group it is more than 2 percent. The result is attributed to the fact that yellow soybean juice is low in calcium and sodium, higher in vitamin B-1 and niacin with more water intake, which contributes to the lowering of blood pressure and increased urination.

Remarks: Yellow soybean sprouts are cool and sweet. They are used to relieve a cough with discharge of yellow mucus and to promote urination.

Black Soybean

*Edema, beriberi, jaundice, rheumatism, muscular cramps, lockjaw,
drug poisoning.*

Description: neutral; sweet; promotes blood circulation and water passage;
counteracts rheumatism; detoxicates; affects the spleen and kidneys.
Applications: Boil 5 g fresh black soybeans in water as 1 dosage, 3 times a day;
or boil until soft, then add sugar and salt as seasonings. Eat at meals; or fry
and grind into powder. Take 1 large teaspoonful of the powder each time,
dissolved in water, twice a day to relieve cough, kidney disease, and peritonitis.
• Regular consumption of black soybeans at meals promotes urination, relieves muscular cramps, and rheumatism and pain in the knees.
Experiment: An experiment on rats indicates that black soybeans produce
effects that resemble a female sex hormone and the effects of an antispasmodic
on the small intestine equal to 37 percent of those produced by papaverine
hydrochloride.

Soybean Oil

Gastric ulcer, duodenal ulcer, intestinal obstruction.

Description: hot; pungent and sweet; lubricates the intestines.
Applications: Prepare 1 teaspoonful of soybean oil and add a few drops of
lemon juice. Drink it on an empty stomach first thing in the morning; gradually
increase the dosage to 5 or 6 teaspoonfuls each time to cure gastric ulcer,
duodenal ulcer, and intestinal obstruction.
Remarks: Soy sauce (a product of soybeans) can promote digestion and it can
also be used as an external remedy to heal burns. But an excessive consumption of soy sauce will cause a cough and thirst and also is not recommended for people with jaundice.

Wheat Bran

*Stomatitis, oral herpes, rheumatism, beriberi, discharge of urine
containing blood.*

Description: cool; sweet; affects the stomach.
Clinical report: A treatment of diabetes: steam 60 percent wheat bran and 40
percent all-purpose flour; add an adequate amount of vegetable oil, eggs and
vegetables. Eat at meals to relieve diabetes. The proportion of wheat bran
decreases as conditions improve. No drugs or nutritional supplements are

given in this treatment. Among the 13 diabetes cases treated, blood sugar dropped to below 140 mg percent in 3 cases and to 180 mg percent in 7 cases; after treatment (which lasts from 4 days to 98 days), sugar in the urine changed from + + + + or + + + to negative in 10 cases; but in general, sugar in the urine changed to negative within 1 month along with the disappearance of neuritis associated with diabetes.

Whole Wheat

Hysteria in women, diarrhea, burns.

Description: cool; sweet; used as a heart tonic and a kidney tonic; affects the heart, spleen, and kidneys.
Applications: Boil 30 g whole wheat kernels with 10 g licorice and 5 red dates in water. Eat once a day to cure hysteria in women. This is a time-honored recipe frequently used in Chinese medicine for hysteria in women.
• Fry wheat until charred and grind into powder to mix with oil for external applications to relieve burns.
Remarks: The grains that float on the water are used as an important Chinese remedy for the above symptoms.

Job's Tears

Diarrhea, rheumatism, muscular twitching, difficulty in movements of joints, edema, beriberi, lung diseases, whitish vaginal discharge.

Description: cool; sweet and light flavor; detoxicates; used as a spleen tonic and a lung tonic; diuretic; affects the spleen, lungs, and kidneys.
Applications: Boil an equal amount of Job's tears, peanuts, and brown sugar. Drink as tea to relieve edema, promote urination, and tone up the stomach.
• Boil 40 g Job's tears to be divided into 2 dosages for consumption twice a day, for 10 days, as a treatment program to relieve flat wart and common wart.
Clinical report: For the treatment of a flat wart: Cook 60 g fresh Job's tears with husked rice in water. Eat it once a day until recovered. Among the 23 cases treated for 7 to 16 days, 11 cases recovered completely, 6 cases showed no clear results, and 6 cases had no results; the majority of patients showed some reactions during the periods between the beginning of treatment and disappearance of the skin rash, including enlargement of the wart focus, which turned red with increased inflammation; but as treatment continued for several days, the damaged focus became dry and desquamative until completely gone.

Remarks: Job's tears is reported to inhibit the growth of and destroy cancer cells. For example, according to a report in the first issue of Jiangsu Chinese Medical Journal (1962), a patient suffering from throat cancer was treated with Job's tears in the hospital, because the cancer was located in the deep region of the throat, which was rather difficult to be treated by surgery. The patient was treated with Job's tears every day, and the treatment produced significant effects within 2 months; the patient recovered completely within 6 months.

Sunflower Seed
Constipation, diarrhea with discharge of blood.

Description: warm and neutral; sweet and light flavor; stops diarrhea; facilitates eruption of rash in measles.

Applications: Crush 30 g sunflower seeds (with shells removed); add 1 cup boiling water and an adequate amount of honey and stir. Drink in the morning and evening to cure constipation.

• Crush 30 g sunflower seeds; add 30 g rock sugar and some water; boil over low heat for 1 hour. Drink 1 cup each time, 3 times a day, to cure diarrhea with discharge of blood.

• Crush 5 g sunflower seeds and make tea. Drink twice a day, to promote eruptions in measles.

• Crush 30 g sunflower seeds with shells, add 30 g rock sugar and boil over low heat for half an hour; drink twice a day to cure ringing in the ears.

Experiment: A normal person consuming unrefined sunflower oil on an empty stomach will temporarily increase the level of their cholesterol; and young women using sunflower oil for cooking for 7 days will slightly lower their levels of cholesterol.

Cottonseed
Impotence, falling of testes, enuresis, hemorrhoids, prolapse of anus, vaginal bleeding and discharge, night sweat.

Description: hot; pungent; warms up kidneys; arrests bleeding; used as a tonic.

Applications: Prepare 300 g cottonseeds and fry with a few teaspoonfuls rice wine; separately fry 100 g chive seeds; grind into powder. Take 10 g with wine on an empty stomach once a day to cure impotence.

• Boil 10 g cottonseeds in 1 glass water over low heat until water is reduced by half. Drink as tea on an empty stomach once a day to cure night sweat.

Remarks: Cottonseed oil is hot and pungent. It may be used externally to relieve boils, tinea, and frostbites. An experiment on chicks shows it can elevate the level of blood fat more than corn or sunflower oil.

Black Sesame Seed

Constipation, dry skin, grey hair, shortage of milk secretion.

Description: neutral; sweet; used as a liver tonic and a kidney tonic; affects the liver and kidneys.

Applications: Fry 15 g black sesame seeds; add some salt. Eat it to increase milk secretion.

• Soak 1 cup rice for a few hours; drain and crush the rice; boil it with 1 cup black sesame seeds in water to make soup. Drink the soup at meals to correct constipation.

Sesame Oil

Constipation due to dryness, ulcers, cracked skin, scabies and tinea.

Description: cool; sweet; detoxicates; lubricates dryness; promotes bowel movements; produces muscles.

Applications: Add a few drops of sesame oil in cooking to relieve constipation.

• Apply sesame oil externally to the affected region and massage it repeatedly to relieve rheumatic pain and fatigue.

Clinical report: For the treatment of chronic simple rhinitis: Cook sesame oil over low heat until boiling. Use as nose drops; apply 2 to 3 drops on each side each time, gradually increasing to 5 to 6 drops, 3 times a day. Among the 63 cases treated, 52 cases showed significant improvements, 3 cases showed progress or improvements, 8 cases showed no effects. Treatment duration ranges from 10 days to 3 months.

8

Meats, Milk, Seafoods, Poultry, and Eggs

Beef

Underweight, diabetes, edema.

Description: neutral; sweet; used as a spleen, stomach, energy, and blood tonic; affects the spleen and stomach.

Applications: Eat regularly concentrated beef soup to relieve chronic diarrhea and prolapse of anus caused by chronic diarrhea.

• Mix together 1,000 g beef, 10 g ground black pepper, 5 g dried orange peel powder; add 1 cup fresh ginger juice and an adequate amount of salt; marinate for 2 hours; cook the beef. Eat at meals to improve the conditions of stomach and stimulate the appetite. To make ginger juice, grate fresh ginger and boil it in water.

Remarks: Beef kidney is used as kidney tonic to improve sexual capacity and to cure temporary and permanent impotence in men; cut a kidney into small pieces to boil with one bowl of rice, and when the kidney is cooked, add five green onion white heads.

• Beef liver is neutral and sweet, is used as a liver tonic, and to sharpen the vision and relieve glaucoma and night blindness.

Lamb or Mutton

General weakness, underweight, abdominal pain, lumbago.

Description: Warm; sweet; used as an energy tonic and to warm up the internal region; affects the spleen and kidneys.

Applications: Cook lamb or mutton with garlic and eat at meals to strengthen erection of the penis and also to relieve upset stomach in men and women.
• Boil 500 g mutton with 1 bowl rice and 1 glass papaya juice; season with sugar and salt. Drink to cure lumbago and beriberi.
Remarks: Mutton can warm the internal region, and for that reason, it is not recommended for people with a hot physical constitution; moreover, mutton is very fatty, not recommended for people with a high level of blood fat.
• Mutton is beneficial for weak and underweight people. Since it may not be easily digested, the quantity eaten each time should be limited.
• Sheep's milk is warm and sweet, is used to lubricate dryness and to relieve fatigue, underweight, diabetes, and vomiting of acid.
• Sheep's liver is cool, sweet and bitter, is used as a liver tonic and to sharpen vision and to relieve glaucoma and night blindness.
• Sheep's kidney is warm and sweet, is used as a kidney tonic and to strengthen sexual capacity and erection of the penis.

Milk

Cow's milk for upset stomach, difficulty swallowing, diabetes, constipation; human milk for fatigue, skinniness, diabetes, difficulty swallowing, dry stools.

Description: Cow's milk—neutral; sweet; pushes downwards; is used as a lung and stomach tonic; and is used to produce fluids and lubricate the intestines; affects the heart, lungs, and stomach. Human milk—neutral; sweet and salty; is used as a blood tonic and to lubricate dryness; affects the heart, lungs, and stomach.
Applications: Boil 1 glass cow's milk in 4 glasses water over low heat until water is reduced to 1 cup. Drink it slowly on an empty stomach to improve physical conditions after a prolonged illness.
• Mix 1 glass cow's milk with half a glass fresh chive juice and 3 teaspoonfuls fresh ginger juice; heat in a small pan. Drink to relieve an upset stomach.
• Mix equal amounts of cow's and sheep's milks. Drink the milk as a substitute for tea or juice to improve the physical condition of diabetes patients and frequent urination.
Clinical report: For treatment of electric ophthalmia by human milk, squeeze fresh human milk directly into a sterilized bottle or sterile eyedrop bottle; apply 2 to 3 drops on the bulbar conjunctiva of the lateral angle of each eye at 5- to 15-minute intervals; close the eyes and rest for a while. In general, discomfort or pain will disappear or decrease within 8 to 16 hours with neither side effects nor discomfort.
Remarks: Cow's milk is not recommended for people with diarrhea or mucous discharge.

Duck

Hot sensations, cough, edema.

Description: neutral; sweet and salty; facilitates water passage and heals swelling; affects the lungs and kidneys.

Applications: Cook a duck with suitable quantities of ham. Eat at meals to relieve diarrhea, particularly chronic diarrhea after childbirth.

• Place 4 to 5 garlic cloves inside a prepared duck; simmer duck in water until very soft. Eat the duck and garlic and drink the soup without salt to relieve chronic nephritis and edema.

Remarks: Duck is good for hot symptoms, such as the presence of internal heat. But it may not be easily digested and is considered bad for hemorrhoids.

• Duck egg is cool and sweet, is used to reduce heat in the lungs and also to relieve cough, sore throat, toothache, and diarrhea.

• Lime, salt, and other ingredients may be used to preserve duck egg to make preserved duck egg, which has a cold energy and pungent and sweet and salty flavors; eat 2 to 3 preserved duck eggs every day (with sugar and vinegar, if desired) to relieve hypertension; or eat 2 preserved duck eggs to check diarrhea and to relieve a hangover. Preserved duck eggs are available in most Chinese food shops.

Chicken

Underweight, poor appetite, diarrhea, edema, frequent urination, vaginal bleeding and discharge, shortage of milk secretion after childbirth, weakness after childbirth.

Description: warm; sweet; used as an energy tonic; warms up the internal region; affects the spleen and stomach.

Applications: Cut up a chicken and remove the skin; pat dry with a paper towel; heat and lightly oil a fry pan; drop chicken cubes into the pan, stirring constantly; add a little vegetable oil and 5 slices fresh ginger and continue to stir-fry for a while. Add 1 cup water and 1 cup rice wine; continue to cook for about 20 minutes; add more rice wine, if desired. Eat at meals to alleviate fatigue and increase milk secretion of lactating mothers.

• Cup up a chicken and remove the skin; wash chicken cubes with rice wine and place the cubes in a fry pan; stir-fry until dried. Steam the chicken cubes with 20 g longans for 3 hours until reduced to half a cup of pure chicken and longan soup. Drink the strained soup (without eating the chicken or longans) to relieve neurasthenia and forgetfulness. This is an expensive recipe; dried longans are available in most Chinese foods shops.

Remarks: Chicken liver is slightly warm and tastes sweet; it acts on the liver and kidneys, is used as a liver and kidney tonic, and also for such symptoms as blurred vision, malnutrition in children, and habitual miscarriage.

Chicken Egg

Dry cough, hoarseness, pink eyes, sore throat, quickening, diarrhea, burns.

Description: neutral; sweet; used as a blood tonic; lubricates dryness.

Applications: Egg may be eaten fresh or mixed with hot water; or use a mixture of egg white and yolk for external applications.

• Break an egg into a cup and mix with a few teaspoonfuls rice wine. Drink it to relieve heart pain in pregnant women.

• Boil 20 chicken eggs in their shells until fully cooked. Crush the eggs, including the shell; boil the eggs again in water with 500 g black soybeans for 2 or 3 hours until the eggs and beans are thoroughly mixed and become black; remove and discard the black soybeans. Store the eggs in a container until needed. Peel the eggs and eat 2 to 3 warm eggs each time, once a day, for as long as necessary, to sharpen vision and correct blurred vision.

Clinical report: For treatment of neurodermatitis and psoriasis, sterilize 2 chicken eggs with alcohol and place in a jar slightly larger than the eggs; add vinegar to cover the eggs and seal; set aside for 7 days. Break the eggs and pour the egg white and egg yolk into another sterilized jar and seal the jar. Use a cotton ball to rub the egg on the affected region for 1 to 2 minutes each time, several times a day; the treatment should continue without interruption. In general, scales begin to fall off after a number of treatments; severe itching either improves or stops completely. If treatment continues, then the focus of the skin ailment will gradually be reduced in size; but if treatment is interrupted at this point, symptoms will recur. The longer the history of symptoms, the longer the treatment needed. Among the 12 cases of neurodermatitis treated, 9 cases recovered completely and 3 cases improved; among the 5 cases of psoriasis treated, 2 cases recovered completely and 3 cases improved.

Chicken Egg White

Sore throat, pink eyes, cough, diarrhea, burns.

Description: cool; sweet; detoxicates; lubricates the lungs; cools hot sensations; considered beneficial to the throat.

Applications: Boil a chicken egg and remove it from the water as soon as it starts to boil; make a hole in the shell and slowly suck the white through the hole to lubricate the throat, once a day, for 3 or 4 months to relieve sore throat, hoarseness, and loss of voice, and to protect the throat in professional singers.

• Mix egg white with rice wine and use the mixture to wash the affected region to heal burns and skin ulcers.

• Mix egg white with 3 teaspoonfuls rice vinegar. Drink it to resume menstruation after childbirth.

Clinical reports: For a treatment of burns, place a chicken egg in 75 percent alcohol and sterilize for 15 minutes; open 2 holes on 2 ends of the egg using a sterile instrument and let the egg white flow into a sterilized container. After debridement (cut off blisters, if any), use a sterilized cotton ball to apply egg white to the burned areas for 2 to 3 times on the first day. In general, a yellowish crust will form on the wound within 6 to 15 hours; by this time, the pain will decrease and the secretion of fluids either ceases or decreases. If the crust forms incompletely, with cracks, apply egg white again until it forms properly and completely. If, however, suppuration occurs under the crust (mostly seen in third degree burns), cut the crust open and incise the pus thoroughly, and then apply egg white again. When burns involve a large area, a lamp may be used to maintain the desired temperature (25 and 31 degrees C). Among the 100 plus patients treated, the majority of patients with first degree and second degree burns (involving areas less than 10 percent) recovered within 10 days; the remaining patients recovered within 12 to 31 days. The majority of patients with first and second degree burns (involving areas between 10 to 20 percent) recovered within 7 to 20 days while the minority recovered within 37 to 60 days. It takes longer for patients to recovered in cases of severe second and third degree burns with areas over 30 percent and complications.

• A report on treatment of infections on the body surface shows that egg white relieves pain, heals inflammation, and prevents suppuration by external applications; and in case of suppurated regions, egg white is found to control inflammation and localize it. Among the 36 cases treated, the patients with smaller areas infected recovered within a single application; the patients with larger areas recovered within 3 to 4 applications. The method of application is similar to the one used in burns.

• A clinical report on the treatment of cervical erosion indicates the method of applications is similar to burns. Use a cotton ball to apply egg white to the erosive areas and then push the cotton ball filled with egg white into the cervix to be removed next day. Each treatment program lasts 3 to 5 days; a second program continues if no results are obtained, and treatment stops during the menstruation period. Among the 32 cases treated, 18 cases recovered and 7 cases improved with 7 cases interrupted. It is indicated that those with bleeding show best results; in addition, the 7 cases treated for cervicitis and vaginitis (developed after childbirth) recovered completely.

• A clinical report on the treatment of otitis media purulenta shows that a mixture of equal quantities of egg white and sesame oil produce satisfactory results when used as ear drops.

Chicken Egg Yolk

Insomnia, muscular twitching, vomiting of blood, hiccupping, diarrhea, miscarriage, burns, hepatitis, malnutrition in children, eczema.

Description: neutral; sweet; used as a blood tonic; and to lubricate dryness; affects the heart and kidneys.

Applications: Swallow a few egg yolks to relieve acute vomiting.

• Mix fresh egg yolk with milk and let children drink it to stop convulsions.

Clinical reports: For treatment of burns use egg-yolk oil after filtration and high-pressure sterilization. Apply the oil to the areas of burns after debridement; exposure is preferred. In more than 100 cases treated for first and second degree burns with small and medium areas, all of them showed good results and no secondary infections occurred. After application of egg-yolk oil, the patients feel cool with decreased pain and effusion of fluids and quicker crusting (which falls by itself) with either no scars or only obscure scars.

• To make egg-yolk oil, boil about 5 to 10 eggs until hard-cooked. Remove the yolks and mash them thoroughly. Fry the yolks in a pan over high heat, stirring constantly, until they gradually turn very dark and close to black, as if the oil is about to flow out; use a clean cloth to wrap the yolks and squeeze out the oil. Apply the oil to burns.

• A report on the treatment of varicose ulcer (stasis ulcer): use the same method as in burns to extract the egg-yolk oil; clean up the affected areas and then apply flat cotton bandage soaked in the oil to the affected region; change the dressing every other day or once every 3 days until recovery.

Remarks: One source indicates that boiled egg yolk may be used to quit smoking.

Chicken Eggshell

Stomachache, gastritis, rickets in children, various types of bleeding, ceruminosis (excessive buildup of earwax).

Description: checks gastric acid; arrests bleeding.

Applications: Crush an eggshell into powder; dissolve 7 g of the powder in rice wine. Drink this amount each time, twice a day, to relieve upset stomach.

• Bake eggshell until dried and crush into powder (the finer, the better). Take 4 g each time with warm water before meals, 3 times a day, to reduce excessive gastric acid, and gastric and duodenal ulcers.

• Break 12 large chicken eggs and mix thoroughly; add 500 g rock sugar and 500 g rice wine; boil until charred and yellowish. Eat a large spoonful each time before meals, 3 times a day, to relieve gastric spasms.

Clinical reports: A clinical report on the treatment of malnutrition in children (56 cases) and rickets (139 cases) and twitching of hands and feet (10 cases) shows that all except 9 cases of chronic indigestion recovered completely within 20 days to 3 months. The treatment: Wash an eggshell and dry it thoroughly; grind it into powder and sieve it (the finer, the better); administer .5 g each time to a 1-year-old child, 1 g for children up to 2 years old, twice a day.

• A clinical report on the treatment of various kinds of bleeding: Simply apply the powder (as made above) to the affected areas with standard precautions of sterilization; the 600 cases treated for traumatic bleeding by this method did not develop suppuration. For the treatment of coughing up blood, vomiting blood, nosebleed, and discharge of blood from anus, apply 6 g of the fine powder with some salt and vitamin C. Administer orally 3 times a day for 2 to 7 days. It is also reported that taking the powder dissolved in water (2 g each time, 3 times a day) relieves allergic skin rash, urticaria, bronchial asthma, excessive stomach acid, and bad breath.

Fresh Ham

Diarrhea, nervousness, poor appetite.

Description: warm; salty; used as a spleen tonic; stimulates the appetite; produces fluids; pushes downwards.

Applications: Boil ham in water with red pepper to make soup; skim off and discard the floating fat. Drink the hot soup to relieve hiccupping and abdominal pain that has lasted for 3 to 4 days.

• Boil 200 g ham in water over low heat for a full day until extremely tender; discard the fat from the surface. Drink as soup to relieve chronic diarrhea.

Pork

Diabetes, underweight, dry cough, constipation.

Description: neutral, sweet and salty; used to lubricate dryness; affects the spleen, stomach and kidneys.

Applications: Boil 500 to 1,000 g pork; skim off and discard the floating fat. Drink the soup to relieve dry cough and constipation.

• Cut up 100 g lean pork (red meats) to boil in water with 100 g Job's tears over low heat for 2 hours. Eat it at meals to moisten the skin; this is considered a good remedy for dry skin.

Remarks: Pork liver is warm, sweet and bitter, acts on the liver and is used as a liver and blood tonic, sharpens the vision, and is considered beneficial to night blindness, pink eyes, edema, and beriberi.

• Pork kidney is neutral and salted; used to relieve lumbago, edema, seminal emission, night sweat, and deafness in the elderly.
• Lard is cool and sweet; lard detoxicates, is used to lubricate dryness, and is considered good to eat for difficult bowel movements, dry cough, and cracked skin.

Abalone

Hot sensations, cough, vaginal bleeding, vaginal discharge, urinary strains, glaucosis, cataract.

Description: neutral; sweet and salty; detoxicates; sharpens vision.
Remarks: Abalone is difficult to digest.

Carp

Common carp for edema, beriberi, jaundice, cough, and shortage of milk secretion; grass carp for headache and rheumatism; gold carp for weak stomach, poor appetite, dysentery, discharge of blood from anus, edema, urinary strains, and ulcers.

Description: common carp—neutral, sweet, pushes downwards, facilitates water passage, promotes milk secretion, and heals swelling, acts on the spleen and kidneys; grass carp—warm and sweet, acts on the spleen and stomach; gold carp—neutral and sweet, used as a spleen tonic, facilitates water passage, acts on the spleen, stomach, and large intestine.

Mussel

Night sweat, lumbago, impotence, vomiting of blood, vaginal discharge, goitre.

Description: warm; salty; increases the energy of kidneys and liver; cures simple goitre; affects the liver and kidneys.
Applications: Bake 100 g mussels and grind into powder. Grind into powder 10 g dried orange peel. Mix the two powders with honey. Dissolve 3 teaspoonfuls in water each time, 3 times daily, to cure insomnia and dizziness.
• Use rice wine to wash mussels and cook with chive. Eat to cure lumbago and to counteract cold sensations in the lower abdomen in women.
• Boil 10 g mussels with 30 g celery. Eat at meals to lower blood pressure.

Clam

Saltwater clam for edema, mucous discharge, goitre, vaginal discharge, hemorrhoids; freshwater clam for vaginal bleeding and discharge, pink eyes, eczema, and hemorrhoids; saltwater clamshell powder for diabetes, edema, goitre, and hemorrhoids; freshwater clam saliva for diabetes, pink eyes, and burns; freshwater clamshell powder for cough with mucous discharge, stomachache, hiccupping, vomiting, whitish vaginal discharge, eczema, swelling.

Description: Sea (saltwater) clam—cold, salty, acts on the stomach, promotes water passage, eliminates mucus, and softens hardness; freshwater clam— cold, sweet and salty, detoxicates, sharpens the vision, acts on the liver and kidneys. Sea clamshell powder—cold, salty, promotes water passage, softens hardness, eliminates mucus, acts on the lungs and kidneys; river clam saliva— sharpens vision; freshwater clamshell powder—cold, salty, eliminates mucus, and dries dampness, acts on the lungs, liver, and stomach.

Applications: Sea clamshell may be baked and ground into very fine powder to make sea clamshell powder. Freshwater clamshell may be washed clean (with the black skin removed) and ground into powder or baked and ground into powder to make freshwater clamshell powder. Apply saltwater clam's saliva externally to the affected region to relieve itching and pain and swelling of the vaginal orifice.

• Crush a few garlics to mix with clamshell powder and make into tablets of a normal size. Take 10 tablets with warm water each time, once a day, to relieve edema in weak persons.

• Mix clamshell powder with lard for external application to the affected region to relieve burns.

• Mix fine clamshell powder with an equal amount of raw licorice powder, take 7 g each time with warm water, twice a day, to cure gastric ulcer and excessive gastric acid.

• Regular consumption of clam meat at meals relieves lymphadenitis scrofula in the neck and goitre.

• Cook clam with chive. Eat at meals to relieve pulmonary tuberculosis and night sweat.

• Boil 30 g fine clamshell powder with 4 g outer layer of peanuts and 6 red dates to make concentrated soup. Drink the soup once a day to relieve nose-bleed, bleeding from gums, and purpura hemorrhagica.

• Roast a whole freshwater clam until its outer part is charred and the inner part becomes yellow-brown with its original shape remaining intact; grind into fine powder and mix with sesame oil for external application to relieve eczema in infants.

Clinical report: For treatment of gastric and duodenal ulcers, fry freshwater clamshell powder in a bronze fry pan (or any earthenware fry pan) until it becomes yellow-brown with the fishy smell gone; strain it before using. Take 1 to 2 g each time mixed with warm water, once every hour during the daytime, 12 to 14 times a day, for 4 to 8 weeks. Among the 41 cases treated from 14 to 79 days, 28 cases showed disappearance of pain in the upper abdomen, and 7 cases a decrease, 23 cases showed disappearance of pressure pain in the upper abdomen (pain that occurs on pressure by hand) and 6 cases a decrease; 21 cases had a follow-up X-ray examination, which indicated disappearance of the niche in 9 cases, disappearance of deformity in 1 case, and a reduction in the size of the niche in 6 cases.

Oyster and Shell

Oyster for insomnia, stress, and nervousness; oyster shell for excessive perspiration, night sweat, premature ejaculation, vaginal bleeding and discharge, tuberculosis of lymph node, goitre.

Description: Oyster—neutral, sweet and salty, used as a blood tonic; oyster shell—cool, salty, obstructive, checks excessive perspiration and premature ejaculation, softens hardness, acts on the liver and kidneys.
Applications: Eat 15 to 25 oysters at meals to cure tuberculosis of the lymph node and goitre; or use oyster sauce as seasoning if fresh oyster is not readily available.
• Crush oyster shell into powder and wrap 15 g of the powder in a cloth. Boil in 3 cups water over low heat until the water is reduced to 1 cup. Drink as tea before a meal, once a day, to relieve excessive gastric acid; or grind the shell into very fine powder and take 3 g of the powder, each time with warm water, 3 times a day.
Clinical report: For treatment of night sweat in pulmonary tuberculosis, boil 20 g oyster shell in 500 ml water until the water is reduced to 200 ml. (Sugar may be added, if desired.) Divide into 2 dosages and drink in the morning and in the evening for a few consecutive days. After the night sweat stops, the treatment continues for another 2 to 3 days to stabilize the effects. Herbal therapy may be used in combination, if no satisfactory results are obtained. In the 10 cases treated, after taking 2 to 3 dosages night sweat disappeared in 7 cases, 3 showed no obvious results, but 2 recovered after being treated in combination with other herbs. No side effects were observed.

Crab

Fractures and dislocations, tinea, skin eruption caused by lacquer.

Description: cold; salty; relieves blood coagulations; cools hot sensations; facilitates recovery of dislocations; affects the liver and stomach.
Applications: Crush a fresh crab to mix with hot broth. Drink it frequently and apply remaining crab to the affected region to restore dislocations; or mix ash

of burned crab with liquor for oral consumption to restore dislocations and heal fractures.

• Crush a fresh crab and apply it to the affected region to relieve lacquer-induced skin eruptions and tinea.

• Bake a crab until charred and grind into powder and mix with rice wine. Take 10 g of the powder and wine each time, twice a day, to relieve jaundice.

• Roast a few crabs until charred and grind into powder. Take 10 g powder with rice wine each time, twice a day, to relieve hypogastric pain after childbirth.

• Bake 1 male crab and 1 female crab and grind into powder; take the powder with wine all at once to facilitate the healing of breast cancer.

• Wrap a fresh crab in a clean cloth, crush it to squeeze out the juice; apply the juice to the affected region for relief of lacquer-induced skin eruptions, or drink the juice all at once to stop or suppress coughing.

Remarks: A male crab has a long navel while a female crab has a round navel.

• Normally freshwater crabs are used in Chinese diet.

• Crab claw is fairly strong in dissolving blood coagulations, and is not recommended for pregnant women (it can cause miscarriage).

• Crab shell powder may also be used for a variety of therapeutic purposes. To make the powder, bake crab shell and grind into powder. Take 10 g powder with rice wine each time, twice a day, to relieve hypogastric pain after childbirth and acute mastitis.

Shrimp

Fresh shrimp for impotence and dry shrimp for shortage of milk secretion.

Description: warm; sweet; used to increase yang energy.

Applications: Crush 500 g shrimps and mix with hot rice wine. Drink it to increase milk secretion; or drink this with soup made from pork leg to reinforce the effects.

Remarks: Shrimp is bad for men with seminal emission or premature ejaculation.

Eel

Fatigue, vaginal discharge, discharge of stools containing blood and pus, hemorrhoids.

Description: warm; sweet; used as an energy tonic, to counteract rheumatism, and to strengthen the bones; affects the liver, spleen, and kidneys.

Applications: Bake an eel after discarding the internal organs; fry 10 g brown sugar and grind with the eel to make a powder. Take the powder with warm water to relieve chronic diarrhea with discharge of stools containing blood and pus.

• Eat eel at meals to arrest bleeding of internal hemorrhoids.

• Boil an eel in an adequate amount of wine until the wine evaporates; bake the eel, including the skin and bones, and grind into powder. Take 10 g each time with a cup of wine in severe cases, or take 7 g in light cases, to relieve difficulty when swallowing. Follow by drinking rice soup and avoiding meat or emotional disturbances and excessive sex.

Cuttlefish

Cuttlefish for anemia, vaginal bleeding and discharge, and suppression of menstruation; cuttlebone for stomachache, excessive gastric acid, vomiting of blood, discharge of blood from anus, vaginal bleeding and discharge, abdominal pain, suppression of menstrual flow, diarrhea, ulcers, and blisters.

Description: cuttlefish—neutral, salty, used as a blood tonic, sharpens vision, acts on liver and kidneys; cuttlebone—slightly warm, salty, used to facilitate water passage, check acid and skin blisters, arrests bleeding, acts on liver and kidneys.

Clinical reports: For treatment of gastric and duodenal ulcers with cuttlebone, use cuttlebone as the key ingredient; cuttlebone is effective for bleeding and perforation due to ulcers, for checking acid and to arrest bleeding and minimize pain due to ulcers.

• For treatment of asthma, mix 500 g cuttlebone powder and 1,000 g sugar for oral administration. Take 20 g each time for adults or a reduced quantity for children, 3 times a day; in general, the treatment takes effect in 2 weeks. Among the 8 cases treated with a history of 3 to 27 years (all treated many times by Western medicine without results), 7 cases were brought under control and the asthma attacks have not recurred despite many changes in weather and 1 case showed improvements.

Sea Grass

Tuberculosis of the lymph node, goitre, edema, beriberi, pain in the testes.

Description: cold; bitter and salty; softens hardness, eliminates mucus; promotes water passage; reduces hot sensations.

Applications: Boil 20 g sea grass at low heat in 4 cups water until water is reduced to 2 cups. Drink 1 cup each time, twice a day, to relieve tuberculosis of the lymph node and goitre, and to prevent hypertension and arteriosclerosis.

• Boil 50 g sea grass with 20 g fried orange seeds and 15 g fried caraway seeds in water. Drink the soup once a day to relieve swollen testes.

Experiments: One experiment shows that sea grass extract can be used as an anticoagulant; another experiment on rats indicates various kinds of sea grass can lower cholestrol in the serum and internal organs; another experiment on dogs and rats shows that when large dosages (.75 g per kilogram) are used, sea grass can lower blood pressure for a prolonged period of time; but smaller dosages will temporarily elevate blood pressure.

Remarks: One source indicates that sea grass can inhibit appetite and cause weight loss. See Kelp for effects on the thyroid gland.

Kelp

Tuberculosis of the lymph node, goitre, hiccupping, difficulty when swallowing, edema, swelling and pain of the testes, vaginal discharge.

Description: cold; salty; softens hardness; facilitates water passage; affects the stomach.

Applications: Regular consumption of kelp at meals relieves goitre; or eat kelp powder with honey.

Experiments: One experiment shows kelp is effective for hypothyroidism due to iodine deficiency; kelp also temporarily inhibits the basal metabolic rate in hyperthyroidism and improves the symptoms for a short duration.

• Another experiment indicates that kelp reduces blood pressure, asthma attacks, and coughing.

Remarks: Kelp is cold and can cool hot symptoms; and it is salty and can soften hardness.

• Prolonged consumption of kelp will cause weight loss. Kelp is not recommended for pregnant women and people with weak digestion.

• To make kelp powder, roast the kelp; dry and grind into powder.

Seaweed

Goitre, edema, beriberi.

Description: cold; salty; softens hardness; eliminates mucus; promotes water passage.

Applications: Prepare 40 g seaweed and wash off the salt; boil it in 2 or 3 glasses water over low heat until the water is reduced by half. Drink to cure simple goitre.

• Boil 20 g seaweed and sea grass each with 5 g caraway seeds in an adequate amount of water over low heat until the water is reduced by half. Drink it to relieve swollen testes.

• Wash seaweed and cut about 1 inch in length; soak seaweed in boiling water 3 times, about 30 seconds each time; strain and eat the seaweed with sugar at meals for 1 month to relieve senile chronic bronchitis.

9

Miscellaneous Foods

Salt

Constipation, bleeding from the gums, sore throat, toothache, carbuncle, cataract.

Description: cold; salty, detoxicates; affects the stomach, kidneys, small and large intestines.

Applications: Brush your teeth with fine table salt in the morning and evening to stop bleeding from gums.

• Mix salt with vinegar and drink it to relieve abdominal pain below the navel.

• Massage the surrounding regions of carbuncle and skin eruptions with salt to relieve itching.

• Drink a cup of salt water first thing in the morning on an empty stomach to relieve constipation.

• Gargle with salt water to prevent and relieve sore throat.

• Lick a little salt with the tip of the tongue before smoking to prevent forming a habit or to quit smoking within 1 month.

• Fry salt until brown; mix it with warm water. Drink the salt water to relieve fish and meat poisoning and abdominal pain due to eating the wrong foods.

• Mix salt with 2 glasses water and wash the affected region to relieve localized dermatitis, skin swelling and itching, and contact skin posion.

• Lick a little salt and let it dissolve in the mouth and slowly swallow it to relieve hiccupping due to improper eating.

Remarks: According to one source, salt can counteract the toxic effects of vegetable alkaloid (this explains why salt can be used to relieve vegetable and herb poisoning).

• According to the *Yellow Emperor's Classic of Internal Medicine*, "Salt travels to the blood, and a person suffering from blood disease should avoid eating excessive salted foods; the kidneys are fond of salted foods." As salty flavor travels to the kidneys first, in taking a kidney tonic, it is customary to add a little salt to reinforce the effects; but salt is bad for edema associated with nephritis.

Royal Jelly

Underdevelopment, loss of weight, poor appetite, hepatitis, neurasthenia, nodular phlebitis, malnutrition, rheumatoid arthritis, anemia, gastric ulcers.

Description: Royal jelly, a modern product not recorded in traditional Chinese diet classics, is now widely used to promote growth, slow down the aging process, and prevent loss of hair; it is produced from a secretion of the worker bees' salivary glands and fermented with honey pollen and other ingredients and specially used as food for the queen bees. This explains why virtually all queen bees are able to live up to 5 years whereas worker bees can live only 2 to 4 months. On top of that, at the height of the laying season, a single queen bee can lay 2,500 to 3,000 ovules that weigh more than the queen bee's own body.

Remarks: Royal jelly is available in tablet form.

Honey

Dry cough, constipation, stomachache, sinusitis, mouth canker, burns, neurasthenia, hypertension, pulmonary tuberculosis, heart disease, liver disease.

Description: neutral; sweet; detoxicates; lubricates dryness; relieves pain; affects the lungs, spleen, and large intestine.

Applications: Steam about half a cup honey. Eat it all at once on an empty stomach, 3 times a day, for 2 to 3 weeks on end, to relieve gastric and duodenal ulcers.

• Mix half a cup honey with warm water and drink once a day to treat hypertension, constipation, stomachache, neurasthenia, heart disease, and coronary sclerosis.

• Drink a cup honey water at bedtime to cure insomnia due to neurasthenia.

• Externally apply honey to the affected region to relieve burns.

• Mix 3 large spoonfuls honey in boiling water. Drink it in the morning and in the evening to relieve insomnia, headache, and anemia; or eat honey at meals with other foods.

• Using a sterilized cotton ball, externally apply honey to the anus to heal cracked skin in hemorrhoids; or externally apply to the ear to relieve swelling of the ear.

• Mix 2 teaspoonfuls honey with warm water. Drink it first thing in the morning on an empty stomach to relieve chronic constipation.

• Mix 1 teaspoonful honey with warm water and drink it 3 hours after meals, 3 times a day, for 5 consecutive days, to relieve hoarseness caused by excessive fatigue but unrelated to common cold, with sufficient rest to produce best results.

Clinical report: For treatment of gastric and duodenal ulcers; among 20 cases treated, the niche disappeared in 15 cases, showed progress in 3 cases (32 days on the average), pain completely disappeared in 18 and pain decreased in 2; pain was gone as quickly as 6 days and within 22 days on the average. The method of treatment: each day, eat a third cup fresh honey before meals, 3 times a day; after the tenth day, increase the quantity of honey to half a cup each day.

• Clinical reports on treatment of other diseases showed good results: For treatment of acute bacillary dysentery, take 150 g honey each day for adults (divide into 4 reduced dosages for children); for treatment of chronic and or temporary constipation in the elderly and in pregnant women, take honey first thing in the morning; for treatment of hypochromic anemia, take 80 to 100 g honey each day, divided into 3 dosages; the results show an obvious increase in blood cells and hemoglobin.

Vinegar

Jaundice, vomiting of blood, nosebleed, discharge of blood from anus, itching in the genital region, fish, meat, and vegetable poisoning.

Description: warm; sour and bitter; disperses coagulations; detoxicates; arrests bleeding; affects the liver and stomach.

Applications: Crush a small piece fresh ginger and mix it with 1 or 2 cups rice vinegar; drink it to correct indigestion caused by an excessive consumption of fish, salads, and fruits.

• Add some vinegar to meats when cooking to promote digestion and stimulate the appetite.

• Cook celery with vinegar as a seasoning to treat hypertension with headache.

• In Chinese folk medicine, when a child suffers from convulsions and faints, with body temperature decreasing rapidly, vinegar is boiled at high heat with the doors closed so that the patient will inhale the vinegar vapor to regain consciousness. The same method may be used to arouse women who faint following childbirth.

• Drink a cup of hot vinegar to relieve pain caused by biliary ascariasis and intestinal ascariasis.

• Combine half a bowl of vinegar, 70 g brown sugar, and 35 g sliced fresh ginger; bring to a boil twice, and strain it. Drink 1 small cup of the liquid each time with warm water, 3 times a day, to relieve itchiness and skin eruptions from allergic reactions after eating fish and crab.

• Soak overnight 10 peanuts in a small cup of vinegar. Drink the vinegar and eat the peanuts the next morning to treat hypertension; repeat for 10 to 15 days as a treatment program.

Clinical reports: A child was suffering from epidemic encephalitis and the Chinese doctor told the patient's father that it was necessary to use lactic acid sterilization; but lactic acid was not readily available. So the father used vinegar as a substitute and obtained good results.

• Once a Chinese food factory reported an epidemic of influenza. All workers in the factory were stricken except the workers in the vinegar division; none of them became ill.

• According to a report from a Chinese food-processing plant, an average 8 percent of the factory workers are sick with respiratory infections yearly; but only 1 percent of the workers in the vinegar division have suffered from respiratory infections each year. Moreover, when the workers in the vinegar division do suffer from respiratory infections, the attack is lighter, too.

• Boil 500 g pork bones and 100 g white sugar in 4 cups vinegar for 30 minutes; strain it. Adults take 30 to 40 ml and children take 10 to 15 ml each time after meals, 3 times a day for 1 month as a treatment program. Chronic patients undergo 2 to 3 treatment programs (except patients with high fever who should not be treated by this method). Among the 3 cases of acute and chronic contagious hepatitis treated, all recovered within 40 to 60 days.

• In Hu Bei Yeecang People's Hospital in China, 51 cases of acute contagious jaundice-type hepatitis were treated with 10 ml rice vinegar and 2 vitamin B-1 tablets. All patients recovered from the illness within an average of 4 days and their poor appetites were significantly improved.

Experiment: In an experiment conducted by the Research Institute of Epidemic Diseases at the Chinese Academy of Medical Science, 200 bacteria colonies were cultured, consisting of 5 bacteria most frequently causing respiratory infections, such as pneumonia, catarrh, and influenza. It was found that all but a few isolated bacteria colonies were exterminated within 30 minutes by vinegar vaporized at 100 degrees C; the same experiment also indicated that vinegar has no obvious bacteria-exterminating power when vaporized below 100 degrees C.

Remarks: Vinegar is called bitter wine in the Chinese language, and vinegar and wine are considered the 2 friends of Chinese herbs. Why? Vinegar and wine are very frequently used to process Chinese herbs, not only to inhibit the side effects of herbs but also to increase their effects.

• Drink between 30 to 50 ml vinegar or more, according to your age, to alleviate the pain caused by biliary ascariasis. This treatment may be repeated until pain is gone. After pain is significantly reduced, apply anthelmintic as usual. Among the 15 cases of biliary ascariasis observed, with a total of 300 to 500 ml vinegar administered in each case, pain stopped completely in 12 cases within 2 days and pain stopped within 3 to 4 days in 3 cases.

Wine

Rheumatism, muscular spasms, chest pain, cold abdominal pain.

Description: warm; sweet, bitter and pungent; promotes blood circulation; expels cold energy; speeds up the effects of herbs; affects the heart, liver, lungs, and stomach.

Applications: Drink a glass of wine to relieve diarrhea due to cold and with the discharge of a clear and long stream of urine, which indicates a cold symptom.

• Mix honey with rice wine and drink it to treat itching all over the body in women.

• Fry 500 g black soybeans until they appear over-fried and begin to crack. Place in an earthenware pot and pour 2 to 4 glasses rice wine into the pot; let it cool and strain it. Drink a cupful each time, twice a day, to heal numbness and pain in the joints, rheumatic pain, neuralgia, and anemia.

• Drink 1 glass hot rice wine or grape wine to relieve pain caused by external injuries.

Clinical report: For treatment of simple diarrhea after childbirth, bring 3 glasses rice wine to a boil; add 150 g brown sugar and continue boiling for 2 to 3 minutes; let it cool and drink it all, or divide it into 2 parts to drink 3 to 4 hours apart. Among the 14 cases treated, 10 cases completely recovered. One case recovered naturally after stopping the treatment, 2 cases showed improvements, and 1 case no significant results. Some cases recovered completely within 3 days. Only 1 case complained about light headache during the treatment. No side effects were shown in all other cases.

Remarks: There are basically 2 kinds of wine used in Chinese herbal therapy— rice wine (also called yellow wine) and hot wine (also called white wine or fire wine). Yellow wine contains only 10 to 20 percent alcohol; white wine contains a much higher alcohol level. White wine is usually used to manufacture medicated herbal wine. Yellow wine is suitable for drinking with Chinese meals.

• Wine is sometimes considered more harmful than beneficial, because many people have a tendency to become intoxicated when drinking wine.

Coffee

Bronchitis, emphysema, cor pulmonale, intoxication.

Description: warm; sweet and bitter; used as a stimulant, heart tonic, and diuretic.

Applications: Drink strong black coffee to relieve intoxication.

• Boil 10 g roasted coffee beans in water. Drink each day to relieve chronic bronchitis, emphysema, and cor pulmonale.

Tobacco

Indigestion, abdominal swelling, headache,
numbness and pain in arthritis.

Description: warm; pungent; toxic; promotes energy circulation, relieves pain; counteracts cold and damp symptoms.

Applications: Boil or squeeze tobacco juice or smoke cigarettes to cure blood coagulations, rheumatic pain, and to warm the body and the womb in women. (Using cigarettes as a form of therapy is a far cry from habitual smoking, which is a form of addiction.)

Experiments: Heavy smokers can develop chronic pharyngitis and other respiratory symptoms; heavy smokers (over 20 cigarettes a day) are 4 to 7 times more susceptible to the attack of bronchitis than nonsmokers.

• Smoking may also be related to lung cancer: Among the lung cancer patients over 45 years old, there are approximately 50 times as many smoking more than 25 cigarettes a day as nonsmokers.

• Smokers are also more susceptible to gastroenteric disorders (such as indigestion, nervous stomach diseases, ulcers, and constipation).

• Heavy smokers may develop headache and insomnia.

• The primary ingredient of tobacco is nicotine, which is very easily absorbed by mucous membranes. When 2 drops are placed on the tongue surface of dogs, they die within 1 to 2 minutes. Nicotine may also be absorbed by the skin surface and cause death.

Remarks: The Chinese people believe that lung cancer may be attributed to excessive heat in the lungs. This may explain why smoking contributes to lung cancer, because tobacco is considered capable of generating the heat that dries the lungs. Thus the lungs become easy targets of cancer when they are hot and dry. For this reason, when a person displays the symptoms of cough and vomiting of blood, smoking could prove fatal.

• Many people gain weight after they quit smoking, which may be due to 2 possible reasons: First, many physicians attribute it to overeating, because when a person quits smoking, he or she needs something else to compensate for smoking, and eating is the easiest candidate; second, according to Chinese medicine, smoking can make the body dry; many overweight persons have a wet physical constitution, and smoking may help them stay slim; when they quit smoking, their body begins to retain water and they gain weight.

• My personal speculation is that if a person has a damp physical constitution (which often means overweight), he or she is less likely to be harmed by smoking; on the other hand, a person with a dry and hot physical constitution is very easily harmed by smoking, and it is wise and urgent for such a person to quit smoking.

Tea

Headache, blurred vision, sleepiness, thirst, indigestion, enteritis, bacillary dysentery, edema in heart disease, herpes zoster.

Description: bitter; sweet; slightly cold; quenches thirst; wakes up the spirits; promotes digestion and urination; affects the heart, lungs, and stomach.

Applications: Grind into powder 10 g tea leaves and 10 g dried ginger. Take one teaspoonful powder with warm water each time, 2 to 3 times daily, to cure acute gastroenteritis.

• Grind tea leaves into powder; dissolve the powder in strong tea and apply externally to the affected region 2 to 3 times daily to cure herpes zoster.

Clinical reports: It is reported that among 168 cases of bacillary dysentery treated by drinking 2 ml strong tea 3 to 4 times daily, 40.6 percent recovered within a few days to a few weeks.

• Strong tea was also used to treat 87 cases of acute enteritis and more than 90 percent of patients recovered within 2 days; the same method was used to treat 12 cases of chronic enteritis. Ten cases completely recovered within 4 to 21 days with stools returning to normal; 2 cases improved to a very significant degree. The method of treatment: Drink 2 to 5 ml of very strong tea 3 to 4 times a day. (Tea leaves are boiled over low heat to make very strong tea, which is different from the normal way of making tea by pouring hot water over tea leaves.)

White Sugar

Dry cough, thirst, stomachache.

Description: neutral; sweet; lubricates the lungs; produces fluids; affects the spleen.

Applications: Boil 3 spoonfuls sugar in 1 glass rice wine over low heat. Drink it to relieve a tight sensation in the abdomen.

• Mix sugar with red dates and chew 2 dates after meals like chewing gum to relieve a dry cough.

• Boil sugar in water to make concentrated syrups to treat stomachache, abdominal discomfort caused by eating fish and crabs, and bad breath caused by eating garlic and onion.

Remarks: Sugar may be boiled and made into the shape of a rock; this is called rock sugar (rock candy) with a neutral energy and sweet flavor. Rock sugar is regarded as the best quality of sugar and is frequently used in combination with other foods in Chinese remedies.

Brown Sugar

Abdominal pain, dysentery, lochiastasis.

Description: warm; sweet; used as an energy tonic; promotes blood circulation; counteracts or eliminates blood coagulations; affects the liver, spleen, and stomach.
Applications: Mix brown sugar with rice wine. Drink it to relieve lochiostasis and faintness after childbirth due to excessive loss of blood.
• Boil brown sugar with 2 plums and drink as tea to relieve dysentery.
Remarks: Both white (granulated) and brown sugar are obtained from the juice of the sugar cane.

Sugar Cane

Vomiting, dry cough, constipation, alcoholism.

Description: cold; sweet; lubricates dryness; promotes urination; produces fluids; pushes downwards; affects the lungs and stomach.
Applications: Drink sugar cane juice to relieve fever, difficult urination, and thirst.
• Mix half a glass sugar cane juice with 3 teaspoonfuls fresh ginger juice. Drink it to relieve vomiting.
• Drink 1 glass fresh sugar cane juice, 3 times a day, to cure light edema during pregnancy.

Hops

Indigestion, abdominal swelling, edema, cystitis, pulmonary tuberculosis, insomnia.

Description: slightly cool; bitter; used as a stomach tonic, digestive, and diuretic.
Applications: Boil 15 g hops in 2 glasses water over low heat until water is reduced by half. Drink once a day to relieve the early stage of pulmonary tuberculosis and low fever in the afternoon.
• Use 4 g hops to make tea every day to relieve neurasthenia, insomnia, and decreased appetite.
Clinical report: On treatment of leprosy, pulmonary tuberculosis, silicosis, silicotuberculosis, tuberculosis of the lymph node, and acute bacillary dysentery, all indicate positive results.
Remarks: One report reveals that Chinese women picking hops in the field normally start to have menstrual flow on the second or third day after they start picking, and they do not experience menstrual pain. The actions of hops and those of a female sex hormone are similar.

10
Preventing and Curing Ailments

INTERNAL CONDITIONS

In China today, diseases are treated either by Western medicine or traditional Chinese medicine or both, depending on the nature of the diseases and the patient's choice. When I visited China in 1983, our bus driver told me of his plans to see a doctor the following day, and I asked him which doctor he wanted to see, a doctor of Western medicine or a doctor of Chinese medicine. He had made an appointment to see the latter, he said. I asked him how he made that choice. Normally, he replied, a Chinese patient relies on the advice of a friend or acquaintance, for that matter, someone who had suffered from a similar disease and had been cured.

Common Cold

• Cook noodles according to the patient's taste, and add 25 g fresh onion white heads and 25 g fresh ginger; mix thoroughly. The patient may begin to perspire afterwards and should stay in bed after eating it.
• Peel and crush 15 g garlic; add 15 ml rice vinegar. Use this mixture the same as the noodles (above).
• Slice 30 g old or fresh ginger and boil in 300 ml water until the water is reduced to 100 ml; add some brown sugar and boil again until the sugar dissolves. Drink the whole thing and stay in bed to perspire.
• Boil 30 g hyacinth beans in water until they break; add 30 g sugar and boil again until the sugar dissolves. After eating, stay in bed to perspire.
• Boil 10 g peppermint and 10 g crushed green onion white heads in water to make tea to relieve headache due to common cold.

• Other foods considered beneficial to common cold are orange peel, peppermint, green onion bulb, and radish.
• Crush 100 g fresh ginger and squeeze out the juice; mix the juice with rice wine and warm in a small pan. Drink the beverage to induce perspiration.
• Fry a few garlic cloves and grind into powder; mix 2 teaspoonfuls of the garlic powder with a little sugar and eat it to relieve cough due to common cold.
• Break an egg into a glass of rice wine and mix with a spoon; warm it over low heat until the egg is half cooked; add some sugar. Drink it as soup to relieve headache and shivering due to common cold.
• Like any other disease, treatment of common cold varies with different symptoms. At the beginning stage, the patient may shiver with cold but without fever, which should be relieved by foods with a warm or hot energy and a pungent flavor (foods with a warm or hot energy will relieve shivering and foods with a pungent flavor will induce perspiration). When the patient with a common cold begins to develop fever, the foods consumed should have a cold or cool energy to reduce the fever (the disease has changed from a cold disease into a hot one); therefore, to reduce the fever the patient should eat foods with a cold or cool energy instead of foods with a warm or hot energy. But the foods with a pungent flavor should still be used to induce perspiration. On the other hand, common cold with a sore throat or any other inflammation should be treated as a hot symptom.

Influenza

• Boil 10 g yellow soybeans in water for 15 minutes; add 30 g parsley and boil it again for 15 minutes. Drink the soup and stay in bed to perspire.
• Slice 250 g fresh radish and soak it in a suitable quantity of vinegar for a few hours. Eat it as salad.
• Put a few slices green onion white heads or garlic in a respiratory mask; inhale for prevention of and recovery from influenza.
• Grate 150 g fresh radish and mix it with honey in a jar. Seal the jar for 1 week. Eat a small cupful each time, 3 times a day.

Diabetes

• Sugar in the urine as one of the most important symptoms of diabetes was included in the Chinese medical classic, *A Collection of Diseases*, by Wang Shou, published in 752. For the first time in Chinese medical history, diabetes was listed among the eleven hundred diseases in the book. The author recommended pork pancreas as treatment for the disease, and had also used a special method of testing sugar in the urine: The patient passed urine on a wide, flat brick to see if ants gathered to collect the sugar. This method of testing urine was more than ten centuries ahead of Richard Thomas Williamson (1862–1937), who invented a test for the same purpose. The Chinese author's treatment using pork pancreas was similar to modern treatment by insulin, a hormone secreted by the beta cells of the islets of Langerhans of the pancreas.

In Chinese medicine, however, thirst, weight loss, fatigue, and sugar in the urine are considered the key symptoms of diabetes. When a patient recovers from any of these symptoms, the diabetes treatment is considered successful.

• Twenty-five diabetes patients were treated at the Canton College of Traditional Chinese Medicine by dried bitter melon slices; each dosage per day consisted of 250 g dried bitter melon slices boiled in water. The levels of their blood sugar taken 2.5 hours after meals, and of their urine sugar taken 24 hours after meals, were both statistically very significant; the same method has subsequently been applied on diabetic rats, which also resulted in a significant decrease in the level of blood sugar; the same report concludes that the effects of dried bitter melon are comparable to those of insulin. It is also suggested that when 100 g fresh clams are boiled in water with the dried bitter melon slices, the results should be better.

• A clinic in the Province of Jiangxi in China reports the treatment of a diabetic patient with good results in which a total of 100 g fresh corn are boiled each time as one dosage. The patient had suffered from diabetes for over 2 years with sugar in the urine, puffiness in the body, frequent urination, and had been treated by Western medicine with no results. Under the treatment by corn the patient had recovered after taking only 4 dosages. Subsequently, another Chinese physician, on reading this report from a medical journal, had used the same remedy to treat a 63-year-old diabetic patient and found it to be equally effective—the patient showed a very significant decrease in the level of blood sugar after undergoing less than 10 treatments. Another clinic in the same province had developed a food cure for diabetes which consists of 60 percent wheat bran and 40 percent wheat powder, mixed with chicken eggs to make a cake remedy (without sugar). At the beginning, the patients were treated with 500 g of this cake remedy each day, with the proportion of wheat bran gradually decreased as symptoms improved. Among the 15 cases treated by this method, the level of blood sugar was tested in 10 cases, among them, blood sugar was reduced to lower than 140 mg per 100 ml blood in 3 cases, and reduced to the level lower than 180 mg per 100 ml blood in 7 cases. All 13 cases showed a general improvement in all other symptoms.

• At the International Symposium on the Effects of Ginseng held in the Soviet Union in 1954, a report indicates that ginseng is capable of lowering the level of blood sugar; and a Chinese physician also points out that according to his experiments, ginseng is capable of reducing the level of blood sugar by as much as 40 to 50 mg per 100 ml blood; such effects can continue for more than 2 weeks after the patient stops taking ginseng. Moreover, in some cases, insulin intake can be reduced while the patient is taking ginseng.

• Chop 50 g fresh potato leaves and 100 g wax gourd; steam over water as a dosage for daily consumption.

• Soak 100 g fresh onion in boiling water for 1 minute; season with a little salt. Eat twice a day.

• Boil 1 cup mare's milk as a daily dosage. Drink the milk twice a day. Mare's milk has a cool energy and sweet flavor; it can lubricate dryness, reduce heat, and quench thirst; it is used for fatigue and diabetes. A Chinese diet classic says, "Mare's milk has the same function as cow's milk, but it is not as fatty as cow's milk; it is effective for reducing the heat of the gall bladder and the stomach, considered beneficial to sore throat, good for the head and the eyes, and also effective for the relief of diabetes."

• According to Chinese herb remedies, pork pancreas has a neutral energy and a sweet flavor; it is used to treat chronic tracheitis, cough, shortage of milk secretion, and emphysema. Boil a pork, beef, or lamb pancreas in water with 200 g yam; season with some salt. Divide into 4 parts. Eat each part once a day for 4 days. Or cut up a pork pancreas and bake until dry over low heat; grind into powder. Take 3 to 5 g in warm water each time, 3 times a day. Or wash the pork pancreas, remove and discard all the white fat, and cut into thin pieces; boil over low heat in water with 20 g corn silk; season with some salt. Eat daily. The use of pork pancreas as an ingredient in a dietary formula to treat diabetes in China was originally published in 1846 in a Chinese diet classic, *New Collected Works of Proven Dietary Recipes*.

• Mix 50 g yam powder with 10 g ginseng powder (readily available in shops). Take 3 times a day, 15 g each time, dissolved in warm water.

• Boil 30 g fresh watermelon peel in 2 glasses water. Drink 1 glass each time, twice a day.

• Soak 100 g mung beans overnight; boil in 3 glasses water over low heat until beans break. Eat as soup in a day.

• Boil 250 to 300 g fresh radish in water with 20 to 25 g abalone. Drink as soup, once every other day. Repeat 6 to 7 times as a treatment program (this is a time-honored recipe in Chinese folk medicine for diabetes).

• Boil 150 g chive (or chive shoots) with 200 g clams and suitable seasoning. Eat in a day. This remedy is also good for excessive perspiration and pulmonary tuberculosis.

Hypertension

• In the Ping-Yang Seaweed Culture Unit in the Province of Zhejiang, China, 110 cases of hypertension were treated by seaweed root powder; in 19 cases (17.3 percent), diastolic blood pressure was reduced by over 20 mm of mercury, and in 65 cases (59.1 percent), diastolic blood pressure was reduced by

10 to 19 mm or to lower than 90 mm of mercury, and systolic blood pressure reduced by more than 20 mm of mercury. The report concluded that the total effective rate of 76.4 percent was achieved and that seaweed roots are waste materials, readily available without any side effects, thus making the therapy both effective and economical.

• In a clinical report, 30 to 40 g dried peanut plants were boiled to make tea as a daily dosage for 2 weeks; patients were instructed to drink the tea from peanut plants on an irregular basis after blood pressure returned to normal. Twenty cases of hypertension were treated by this method; the majority showed improvements within 3 days with a significant decrease in blood pressure (the mean value—systolic pressure was reduced by 29 mm and diastolic pressure by 30 mm of mercury).

• A patient of hypertension in Tianjin, China, wrote to an editor to say that he had been suffering from hypertension with dizziness and constipation for many years but had been unable to find a cure; subsequently, he began to eat 5 bananas every day, which eventually cured his disease.

• A Chinese physician reported a 49-year-old female patient suffered from hypertension with occasional constipation, headache, and dizziness; she had taken honey for 2 months, which reduced her blood pressure to normal and cured her constipation as well.

• There are basically 3 ways to cope with hypertension, according to the Chinese diet system. First, eat more foods that can soften the blood vessels, such as kelp, sea grass, mung bean sprouts, fruits, and others, to prevent arteriosclerosis. Second, use vegetable oils such as sesame, peanut and corn oil, instead of animal fats and oils to reduce the level of cholesterol; and avoid foods with a high cholesterol level, such as egg yolk, liver, and kidneys. Third, eat more foods that can reduce blood pressure, such as celery, hawthorn fruit, banana, and persimmon.

• Wash 500 g fresh celery, and squeeze out the juice; mix the juice with 50 ml honey and warm it in a small pan. Divide and drink twice a day.

• Soak mung beans in water overnight; the next day, boil with an equal amount of seaweed and some rice (for long-term consumption).

• Eat 1 to 2 fresh tomatoes on an empty stomach first thing in the morning for 15 days. Repeat from time to time as a treatment program. This is also good for constipation.

• Cook tomatoes with celery as soup; season with a little salt.

• Chop 750 g water chestnuts and 750 g radishes; squeeze out the juice; mix with a few teaspoonfuls honey. Drink the juice twice a day, half of the portion each time.

• Fry 20 g kelp with 20 black soybeans; boil kelp and soybeans in 3 cups water until water is reduced by half. Eat as soup.

• Regularly eat seaweed, mung beans, hawthorn fruit, clams, and mung bean sprouts.

Kidney Disease

• Wash and peel 300 g old ginger; crush it to squeeze out the juice; soak 50 g red dates in water for half an hour until soft; crush them after peeling and removing the seeds. Combine ginger juice and crushed dates in container; add 100 g brown sugar and steam until they become like a pudding. Eat 3 times a day for 5 days.

• Chinese people in small villages have the habit of eating "watermelon sugar" as a food to treat kidney disease. Slice watermelon (red part only) into thin pieces and cook over low heat; then add a little sugar and strain; after 4 or 5 days, the juice will thicken like honey, which is called watermelon sugar. Eat 1 tablespoonful each time, twice a day.

Nephritis

• Using a sharp knife, make a triangular hole in a 1.5 kg watermelon to remove some flesh; place 70 g peeled garlic cloves inside the watermelon; cover the hole with cut piece of the rind; steam the watermelon with the garlic; and eat the whole thing while hot.

• Boil 30 g dried watermelon peel in water. Drink as tea. Or boil 2 corncobs in water and drink it as tea.

• Eat 1 or 2 fresh cucumbers; or crush the cucumbers to squeeze out the juice. Drink as tea; or boil dried cucumbers in water as soup.

• Prepare a large carp by removing the internal organs; do not scrape off the scales; use a cloth to dry the fish. Boil the carp in water with 1 cup small red beans without salt. Drink the soup, which is also good for edema due to nephritis during pregnancy in women.

• For difficulty when urinating, eat more foods that can promote urination, such as eggplant roots, cucumber, wax melon seeds and peel, corncob, watermelon peel, small red beans, sea grass, lily flowers, radish, black soybeans.

• Avoid fresh garlic, green onion, chive, red pepper, nicotine, alcohol.

Bronchitis

• Crush 500 g unpeeled radish or pear and soak in 2 teaspoonfuls honey for a few hours before eating it.

• In case of hoarseness due to bronchitis, boil some licorice in water over low heat. Eat as soup.

• Clean out a chicken and peel a grapefruit; stuff the grapefruit into the chicken cavity, place in a pan, and add a little water; steam the chicken with the grapefruit inside. Eat the chicken and drink the broth. Repeat this remedy 3 times, once every other week.

• Older patients suffering with chronic bronchitis should be more energetic by eating fish, seafoods and yam.

Bronchial Asthma

• Wash and boil a pumpkin with 2 teaspoonfuls honey in water until the pumpkin becomes extremely soft; use the condensed pumpkin soup to mix with 10 g fresh ginger juice. Boil the new mixture for a few minutes. Drink 1 cupful each time with warm water, 3 times a day.
• Boil together 200 g bean curd, 60 g maltose or honey, and 30 g fresh radish. Eat in 1 day to relieve the symptoms.
• Boil 2 g fennel seed or anise seed, 10 g apricot seed, 5 g dry orange peel, and 8 g seaweed in 3 cups water until the water is reduced to 1 cup. Drink 1 cup as tea each time, 3 times a day.

Tuberculosis of the Lymph Node

• Boil together 50 g dried litchi, 15 g seaweed, 15 g kelp, and 1 teaspoonful wine in water. Eat the mixture in 1 day.
• Boil some noodles in water until half cooked; add 50 g fresh oyster meats and 15 g fresh garlic, crushed; boil again for a few minutes and season with some salt. Eat the entire stew in 1 day.
• Peel 90 g garlic cloves; boil them in water with 2 unshelled duck eggs; when the eggs are hard-cooked, peel them and cook again for a while. Drink the soup and eat the eggs and garlic. (Duck eggs should be used instead of chicken eggs, for duck eggs can tone up yin energy and cool down the lungs.)
• Boil 120 g fresh kelp or 60 g dried kelp with an adequate amount of rice vinegar. Eat it as soup. This is not recommended for people with gastric and duodenal ulcers or excessive stomach acid.

Mumps

• Boil 50 g fresh lily flowers or 20 g dried lily flowers; add some salt. Drink it as soup.
• Crush 10 g peeled garlic cloves in 10 ml rice vinegar for external application to the affected region; or soak 50 g small red beans in water for 30 minutes and crush them for external application to the affected region; or soak 50 g small red beans overnight; boil until tender the next day. Eat it as soup in 1 day.

Contagious Hepatitis

• Boil together 4 cups rice vinegar, 500 g pork spareribs, 125 g brown sugar and 125 g white sugar for 30 minutes or less without adding water. Strain and drink each time as follows: 10 to 15 ml for 5- to 10-year-old children; 20 to 30 ml for 11- to 15-year-olds; 30 to 40 ml for adults; 3 times a day after meals for 1 month as a treatment program; and 2 to 3 treatment programs for chronic patients.

• Wash 100 to 150 g fresh celery and squeeze out the juice; steam the juice with honey. Eat it warm once a day.

Gastroenteritis

• Bake 100 g tea leaves and 50 g fresh ginger; when dry, grind into powder. Take 3 g of the powder each time, 3 times a day, with warm water. This is a good remedy for acute gastroenteritis.

• Boil 50 g hyacinth beans in water as a day's dosage; divide and eat it twice a day. Or bake hyacinth beans until dry and grind into powder. Take 15 g of the powder in warm water each time, twice a day. Another good remedy for acute gastroenteritis.

• Wine made from grapes is considered good for chronic gastroenteritis.

• Mix large pinches of ground nutmeg, ground cinnamon, and a small pinch of ground cloves; divide into 3 equal portions. Take 1 portion in warm water each time, 3 times a day: Good for chronic gastroenteritis and cold stomach.

Gastric and Duodenal Ulcers

• A well-known Japanese physician reported that a German professor at Berlin University used licorice powder to treat patients of gastric ulcers with remarkable results. According to this report in a German medical journal, 38 patients were treated with 20 to 25 g licorice every day for 6 weeks; the gastric ulcers were completely gone in 32 cases, verified by X-ray examination; subjective sensations of stomach discomfort were eliminated in 3 cases. The remaining 3 cases showed no effects, but when subsequently treated by surgery were found to have stomach cancers.

• During the treatment, salt intake should be controlled and patients should be on high-protein and -vitamin diets. The professor pointed out that if a patient of gastric ulcer does not respond to treatment of licorice powder, the possibility of stomach cancer may be indicated. Subsequently, a professor and 2 assistants at Kyushu University in Japan also reported their treatment of licorice powder for 6 Japanese patients of gastric ulcers; the results indicated that abdominal pain and heartburn were completely gone within a week, gastric juices returned to normal, and stools were free of blood within 2 weeks. X-ray examinations a month later verified the patients were completely cured.

This dramatic cure of gastric ulcers, they pointed out, has never occurred in the past except by surgery.

• Soak 50 g fresh peanuts in water for 30 minutes, drain and crush them; bring 200 ml fresh milk to a boil and add the peanuts; again bring to a boil; remove from the heat to cool; add 30 ml honey. Eat it once a day, an hour before bedtime.

• Cut up and crush 50 g unpeeled fresh potatoes; squeeze out the juice and add a suitable quantity of honey to the juice. Drink the juice on an empty stomach first thing in the morning for 20 days. The tomato's sour flavor will be neutralized by the honey.

• Avoid irritating foods (liquor, coffee, red and black pepper, ginger), foods with a cold energy (crab, clam, seaweed, mung beans, wax gourd), and foods with a sour flavor (vinegar, lemon, plum, hawthorn fruits).

• Boil 3 bean curds with 60 g brown sugar in a glass of water for 10 minutes. Drink it as soup. This remedy is recommended for bleeding or vomiting of blood or discharge of black stools caused by gastric and duodenal ulcers.

• Boil 50 g Job's tears and 10 g licorice in 2 cups water. Drink it as soup.

• Boil fresh lotus roots in water over low heat to make a concentrated juice. Drink 1 cup a day for 2 weeks as a treatment program.

Gastroxia (Hyperchlorhydria)

• Take 5 g abalone bone powder with warm water each time, half an hour before meals, 3 times a day. Avoid getting too hungry, too full, or too tired. To make abalone bone powder, wash the bones and bake until dry; scrape the outer layer and grind into powder. Store the powder in a jar.

• Eat some fresh ginger or sweet fruits or strong tea or a few slices of garlic 2 or 3 hours after meals to relieve pain or heartburn.

• Roast oyster shells and grind into powder. Take 2 g of the powder in warm water each time, 3 times a day.

Stomachache

• A Chinese physician reported that he treated 34 cases of cold diseases with remarkable results; these included cold stomachache, vomiting of acid, abdominal swelling, intestinal rumbling, diarrhea, chest pain, cough, and abdominal pain during menstruation in women. The above diseases are classified as cold diseases, because all the patients show 3 basic cold symptoms: dislike of cold as it makes their symptoms get worse, absence of fever, and no sensations of thirst. The remedy consists of 10 to 15 g licorice and dried ginger mixed together as a dosage for one day.

• A Chinese physician reported his successful treatment of 20 cases of cold stomachache. To make his remedy: combine 10 raw black peppercorns, 3 red seeded dates, 5 apricot seeds (from sweet or bitter apricots) and immerse in warm water for 2 days (change water 5 times during that period); drain and crush the 3 ingredients, mix them with a small amount of warm water to make a thick soup. Drink the soup with water for a dosage (reduce for children).

A 75-year-old patient treated in this program who had a 10-year history of stomachache, came to the clinic because his chronic stomachache was triggered by a cold meal the previous evening. His stomachache was gone only 30 minutes after drinking the soup. The Chinese doctor visited him a month later and found the patient in good health.

• Warm ¾ cup fresh milk with 1 teaspoonful fresh ginger juice and a little sugar; drink the whole thing. It's also good for vomiting, belching, and difficulty when swallowing.

• Dissolve 4 g ground cinnamon in a cup of warm water; cover it for 15 minutes. Drink it as tea.

Abdominal Pain

• Boil a few garlic cloves in water with black sugar over low heat. Drink a cupful each time, 3 times a day, after meals.

• Chew a few dried sour plums slowly like chewing gum.

• Consume a large quantity of cooked chives.

Bacillary Dysentery

• In a Chinese clinic, 24 patients of bacillary dysentery were cured by tomato plants. To make the remedy: wash tomato stalks, branches, and leaves of 2 to 3 tomato plants (about 1 kg); boil them in water for 3 hours, and make juice by straining through a clean cloth and squeezing. Drink 1 to 2 cupfuls each time, 6 to 10 times a day.

• Two Chinese hospitals in the Province of Sandong reported that 91 patients, 34 with bacillary dysentery and 57 with enteritis, were treated by a simple remedy with remarkable results. The remedy: charred hawthorn fruits and hyacinth bean flowers; the patients, divided into 3 groups, were treated separately by 3 remedies—charred hawthorn fruits, hyacinth bean flowers, and a combination of the 2 ingredients; 24 cases of bacillary dysentery (83.33 percent) were cured by charred hawthorn fruits alone, 35 cases of acute enteritis (71.43 percent) by hyacinth bean flowers alone. It is also pointed out raw and charred hawthorn fruits do not have significant differences in treatment results, which means that either may be used for the treatment.

• Cut up peeled fresh radishes; add some rice vinegar, and sugar. Eat twice a day.

• Eat steamed potatoes with honey, 3 times a day.

• Place 100 g green tea leaves in 700 ml water; bring to a boil and cook for 20 minutes or until reduced to 75 ml water; remove from heat to cool; add 25 ml white wine. Drink 2 ml each time, 3 times a day.

Chronic Amoebic Dysentery

• Chew 1 garlic clove each time, 3 times a day for 7 days, along with other foods.
• Boil 50 g fresh guava peel in water as a day's dosage.
• The above 2 remedies are not suitable for acute amoebic dysentery.

Roundworms on the Biliary Tract

• A 27-year-old female patient of biliary ascariasis was cured by a formula of 3 ingredients: 15 g licorice, 12 g honey, and 10 g nonglutinous ground rice. To make the remedy, boil licorice in water; then pour the hot licorice juice into the mixture of honey and rice powder. Drink it hot.

When the patient with 10 roundworms was admitted to the clinic, she was in severe pain in the right upper abdomen and vomiting frequently. She was treated by both Western and Chinese medicines for 3 days without results but with severe pain (the doctors refrained from using strong pain killer due to her pregnancy). By taking this remedy, the patient's pain was gone within a day and she recovered completely within 6 days when some Chinese herbs comparable to piperazine were also administered; she gave birth to a boy a few months later.
• Mix 40 ml rice vinegar with an equal amount of warm water for 1 dosage. Drink 3 times a day for 3 days.
• Drink 10 ml fresh ginger juice with warm water each time, once every hour for 4 times; repeat 3 times a day for 2 days.
• Grind 10 black peppercorns; add 100 ml water and boil for 30 minutes. Strain and drink all the liquid each time, twice a day.
• The above 3 recipes may be used alternately; after symptoms are eliminated, piperazine should be used to prevent a recurrence.

Iron-Deficiency Anemia

• Boil 50 g mung beans and 50 g dried red dates in water until the beans break; add some brown sugar. Drink once a day for 15 days as a treatment program.
• Put 100 g sweet or brown rice and 30 g black soybeans in boiling water; simmer until half cooked; add 30 g red dates and continue cooking until well done; add brown sugar as seasoning. Eat once a day.

Macrocytic Anemia

• Wash 150 g spinach; cut up 50 g pork liver. Bring water to a boil; add the spinach and pork liver and boil for a few more minutes; season with salt. Eat once a day until recovery.

• Prepare a pork kidney as you would normally; soak it in warm water for 30 minutes; cut it up in thin pieces and boil the pieces in water. Add salt as seasoning. Eat it once a day or every other day until recovery. (Beef, veal, or lamb kidneys may be used as substitute).

Aplastic Anemia

• Soak 30 g black fungus in water for 30 minutes; drain. Boil the fungus with 30 red dates and some brown sugar. Eat once a day until recovery.

Granulopenia

• Boil 50 g fresh mushrooms; add salt as seasoning. Eat daily until recovery.

Hemophilia

• Eat 50 g unshelled fresh peanuts, including the peanut and skin, 3 times a day for 2 weeks as a treatment program.

Anaphylactoid Purpura (Allergic Purpura)

• Two Chinese physicians reported they cured 6 cases of athrombopenic purpura, including purpura simplex and allergic purpura, by using red dates. For the remedy, wash fresh red dates (or dried ones). Eat 10 dates each time, 3 times daily, until purpura is completely gone.

   No other remedies are used except in one case, which is also given vitamins C and K and benadryl. Purpura disappeared within 2 days in 1 case, 3 days in 3 cases, 7 days in 2 cases, with an average of 4 days. A follow-up visit indicated no recurrence in 5 cases and recurrence in 1 case, possibly caused by premature termination of the treatment. The physician indicated treatment should continue for a few days after purpura is gone, to prevent a recurrence.

• Boil 100 g barley with 15 g red dates in 500 ml water until reduced to 150 ml water. Eat the whole thing as a day's dosage.

• Put 250 g red dates in 1,500 ml water and bring to a boil; crush the dates as soon as they swell; continue to boil for 40 minutes, then drain over a bowl and save the juice. Add 300 ml water to the dates and boil over low heat for 20 minutes; drain it again and save the juice. Boil the reserved juice until reduced to 750 ml. Drink 1 cup of the juice each time, 3 times a day.

• Prepare 30 g peanut shells and 30 g red dates. Boil the 2 ingredients; drain and save the soup. Drink the soup all at once as a day's dosage; repeat for 5 days as a treatment program.

Coronary Atherosclerotic Heart Disease

• Boil 50 g yellow soybeans in water; add salt as seasoning. Eat in 1 day; repeat as often as necessary.
• Boil 30 hawthorn fruits in water; season with sugar and eat this amount each day of the treatment; repeat as often as necessary.

Simple Goitre

• Bake 500 g seaweed and 500 g sea grass until dry; grind into powder. Take 10 g of the powder in warm water each time, once a day.
• Boil 10 g seaweed and 10 g kelp in water. Drink the soup as tea.

Sunstroke

• Boil 50 g hyacinth beans in 500 ml water until reduced to 300 ml; add salt as seasoning. Drink half the cooled juice each time, twice a day and eat the beans.
• Peel a wax gourd weighing about 500 g; crush it to squeeze out the juice; season with salt. Drink it slowly.
• Wash and peel a radish; grate it to squeeze out the juice. Drink it with cold water.
• Slice a bitter melon in small pieces; cook in water as soup or as an ingredient in a recipe.

Alcoholism

• Pour boiling water into a teapot containing 15 g tea leaves; wait for 10 minutes. Drink it all at once.
• Boil 60 g black soybeans in water. Drink it as soup.
• Put 15 g sugar in 30 ml rice vinegar; add a little hot water to dissolve the sugar. Drink it all at once.
• Boil 30 g hyacinth beans in water. Drink it as soup.
• Cut finely 2 g dried orange peel; add 2 sliced seeded plums; boil the peel and plums in 2 glasses water over low heat for 30 minutes; drain over a bowl; add fresh ginger juice and strong tea to the liquid. Drink it as tea.
• Wash 20 g black soybeans; cut open a coconut (saving the liquid) and place the black soybeans in the coconut and close it again; steam the coconut in a bowl for 4 hours; add salt to the coconut liquid.

• Use American or Western ginseng (not Korean or Chinese ginseng, which have altogether different actions) either in soup or in powder form, once a day.

Smoking

• Grate a fresh radish and mix with 2 teaspoonfuls honey. Drink as juice.
• Prepare 100 g fresh bean curd and 50 g black sugar; make a few holes in the bean curds and put black sugar into the holes; steam bean curds. Whenever a person has an urge to smoke, eat a few spoonfuls of bean curds with black sugar inside to quit smoking. This will make the habitual smoker want to vomit on exposure to the smell of tobacco.

FEMALE CONDITIONS AND AILMENTS

Menstrual Disorders

• Prepare 120 g lamb liver, 90 g chives, 1 tablespoon peanut oil, and some light soy sauce. Cut chives and liver as you would in normal cooking. Heat a wok or fry pan over high heat and pour the oil into the pan; add the chives and stir-fry for a short while; drop the liver into the wok and stir-fry again for a short while; season with light soy sauce and cook for a few more seconds. Good for irregular menstruation and vaginal bleeding; also good for vaginal discharge.
• Fry 30 g black fungus over low heat; add a bowl of water and continue cooking; add 15 g sugar as seasoning. Good for excessive menstrual flow that belongs to a hot symptom only. This remedy is not recommended for treatment of excessive menstrual flow due to blood deficiency.
• Scrape and slice 120 g fresh celery and 120 g lotus roots as you would in normal cooking; place a wok or fry pan over high heat and pour 1 tablespoon peanut oil into the pan; when hot, add the celery and lotus roots and stir-fry for 5 minutes before adding salt as seasoning. Good for irregular menstruation and vaginal bleeding of a hot nature.
• Boil 30 g dried ginger in water along with 30 g brown sugar and 30 g seeded red dates. Good for menstrual pain of a cold nature.
• Prepare 24 g fresh ginger, 30 g red dates, and 9 g red pepper. Cut the ginger and pepper as you would in normal cooking; boil the 3 ingredients in 3 glasses water until the water is reduced by half. Drink it hot to relieve cold menstrual pain.
• Cook 60 g black soybeans, 2 unshelled eggs, and 120 g rice wine over low

heat; peel eggs after cooking and then cook eggs again; add rice wine. Eat the eggs and drink the hot soup to relieve menstrual pain due to energy and blood deficiency.

• Boil 5 g cinnamon twigs, 15 g hawthorn fruits, and 30 g brown sugar in 3 glasses water until water is reduced by half; add brown sugar and continue to boil for a few seconds. Drink it hot to relieve menstrual pain due to coldness and blood coagulations.

• Boil 50 g fresh parsley in 3 cups water until the water is reduced to 1 cup; crack 1 egg into the boiling water (the egg coagulates to look like flowers); add some seasoning. Eat it to relieve menstrual pain. This recipe is also good for stomachache and nervous headache.

• Fry a 250-g cuttlefish in vegetable oil with 40 g thinly sliced fresh ginger; season with salt. This is a remedy for relief of suppression of menstruation.

Leukorrhea

• Boil 15 g hyacinth beans, 30 g yam, 60 g sweet rice in 500 ml water over low heat. Drink as soup to relieve whitish vaginal discharge. Or boil 60 g hyacinth beans in water; add some sugar as seasoning. Drink as tea for relief of whitish vaginal discharge. Or, fry an equal amount of hyacinth beans and yam and make tea to stop whitish vaginal discharge.

• Boil 30 g Job's tears in 750 ml water with 30 g seeded red dates and 60 g sweet rice over low heat. Drink as soup to relieve whitish vaginal discharge due to weakness.

• Boil 2 cuttlefish with 250 g lean pork in water; season with salt. Eat it once a day for 5 days as a treatment program to relieve whitish vaginal discharge.

• Boil 10 dried radish leaves in 3 glasses water; add a little salt. Drink the hot soup to induce perspiration, twice a day, for 1 to 2 months to relieve whitish vaginal discharge.

Symptoms Associated with Pregnancy

• Clean a 250-g gold carp as you would in normal cooking; steam it along with 90 g small red beans until the beans are soft. In general, edema during pregnancy should be cured after eating this 5 or 7 times.

• Boil 50 g wax gourd peel and 50 g small red beans in water without adding salt. Drink as tea to relieve edema during pregnancy.

• Prepare 125 g fresh peanuts, 10 red dates, 30 garlic cloves, thinly sliced, and 15 g peanut oil. Heat a wok or fry pan over high heat; pour peanut oil into the wok and stir-fry the garlic; then add peanuts and dates with 1,000 ml water; boil until peanuts are very soft. This dish should produce effects for edema during pregnancy after eating it for 7 to 10 times.

• Steam 9 g grapefruit peel and 12 g Chinese salted brown olives in 600 to

700 ml water until olives are fully cooked. In general, this remedy should relieve morning sickness after eating it 5 to 7 times.
• Boil 15 to 20 g grapefruit peel in water. Drink it as tea to relieve morning sickness.
• Bring 1,000 ml water to a boil over high heat; add 100 g black soybeans and 30 g sliced garlic cloves, and 30 g brown sugar; boil over low heat until the soybeans are fully cooked. In general, edema during pregnancy should be cured after eating this 5 or 7 times.
• Fry 250 g sweet rice with 30 ml of fresh ginger juice until the rice breaks; grind into powder. Take 10 to 20 g in warm water each time, twice a day, to cure morning sickness.
• Bring 60 ml rice vinegar to a boil; add 30 g sugar and stir until dissolved; break the egg into the boiling vinegar. When the egg is cooked, drink the whole thing to relieve morning sickness.
• Fry 1 cup rice bran; then wrap it in a cloth bag or cheesecloth; add water and simmer over low heat; add some sugar, if desired. Drink it as tea to cure beriberi during pregnancy.
• Soak 100 g small red beans overnight; next day, boil in 3 glasses water until beans begin to break. Drink as soup to cure edema and water retention during pregnancy.

Symptoms After Childbirth

• Boil 150 g bean curd with 50 g brown sugar in 3 cups water; add 50 ml rice wine when sugar dissolves. Drink all at once, once a day for 5 days to increase milk supply after childbirth.
• Crush a river crab; boil it with 60 ml rice wine. Eat in 1 day. In general, this dish should produce results in increasing the milk supply following childbirth after eating it 3 to 5 times.
• Prepare 30 g lily flowers and 60 g lean pork as you would in normal cooking; steam the 2 ingredients over high heat until the pork is well done. Eat the whole thing to increase the milk supply after childbirth and also to relieve mastitis.
• Simmer 500 g papaya along with 500 ml rice vinegar and 30 g fresh ginger over low heat for 40 minutes. Drink as tea, twice a day, 1 small glass each time, to increase the milk supply after childbirth and also to relieve lochio-stasis.
• Fry 120 g malt over low heat for a few seconds; add 750 ml water and bring it to a boil and cook until the malt is fully cooked; add 30 g brown sugar. Drink it as soup once a day for 5 to 7 days to stop milk secretion.
• Boil 30 g hawthorn fruits in water until very soft; add 30 g brown sugar. Drink as tea to relieve lochiostasis and blood coagulations after childbirth.
• Fry 500 g black soybeans over low heat until they become half burned, add

350 ml rice wine and marinate overnight. Next day, strain it and drink half a glass of wine each time, 3 times a day, to relieve rheumatic pain after childbirth.
• Eat cracked wheat and brown rice on a regular basis to promote milk secretion.
• Boil 10 g anise seed in water to make soup; add some wine. Drink it to promote milk secretion.

Other Women's Diseases

• Put 1 kg fresh litchis with seeds (or dry litchis in a reduced quantity) in 1 L rice wine; seal the container and put away for 1 week. Drink twice a day, depending on your appetite, to cure prolapse of the uterus.
• Wash and steam a few crabs; when they are fully cooked, add 2 teaspoonfuls rice wine and steam for 1 more minute. Drink the soup and eat the crab with soy sauce to relieve abdominal pain after childbirth.
• Put a grapefruit or its peel in the bathtub while taking a bath; this will give off an aromatic smell, considered good to warm cold sensations in women.
• Steam black soybeans and dry them in the sun; grind into powder; add an equal amount of ground sesame seeds and some honey; drink the 3 ingredients with warm water to cure frigidity in women.

OTHER HEALTH PROBLEMS

Prolapse of the Anus

• Boil 200 g fresh parsley in water. Wash the anus with the liquid once a day.
• Boil fig leaves in water. Use the liquid to wash the affected region or sit in the liquid while taking a bath.

Hemorrhoid

• Fry 250 g clams in some peanut oil; add 10 g sliced fresh ginger and some water and cook until the clams are very soft; add some salt. Eat it on an empty stomach, once every other day, 7 times as a treatment program.
• Eat 1 to 2 bananas with the peel on an empty stomach first thing in the morning.
• Eat 1 to 2 figs on an empty stomach first thing in the morning. Or boil fig leaves in water; use the liquid to wash the affected region or sit in the liquid in the bathtub.
• Steam 60 g dried figs in an adequate amount of water with 100 g lean pork; season to your taste. Eat for as long as a month as a treatment program.
• A Chinese army physician writes a report on his successful treatment of 27

cases of hemorrhoids by a simple remedy of figs. To use his remedy, prepare 10 fresh or dried figs and simmer in 1 L water over low heat for 30 minutes after the water begins to boil; the water should be reduced to about .7 L. Eat 5 figs each time, twice a day; also, repeatedly wash the affected region with the hot cooking water of the figs for 20 minutes. During the treatment, the patient should refrain from eating pungent or hot foods. The history of hemorrhoids among the 27 cured cases is as follows: 3 cases more than 10 years; 7 cases between 6 and 10 years; 17 cases between 1 and 5 years; patients recovered within 12 treatments in 4 cases, within 5 treatments in 9 cases, and within 6 to 11 treatments in 14 cases, with the average being 7.6 treatments.

• Boil 30 g black fungus with 30 red dates over low heat. Eat once a day for 10 days as a treatment program.

• Boil 60 g lily flowers in water with an adequate amount brown sugar. Eat before breakfast for 1 week as a treatment program.

• Peel 2 bananas and steam them with an adequate amount of rock sugar. Eat them twice a day for 1 week.

Mastitis

• See Symptoms after Childbirth.

• Boil 150 g green onion white heads and 60 g malt in 500 ml water for 20 minutes; wrap the onion heads and malt in a clean white cloth. Use hot to rub repeatedly along the breast towards the nipple, particularly in the hard area, until the breast becomes red and soft. This treatment is applicable only in the early stage of acute mastitis prior to suppuration.

Carbuncle

• See the bean remedy under Erysipelas.

• Bake some small red beans and grind them into powder; mix with honey to make an ointment. Apply externally to the affected region until healed; change the dressing as soon as it dries.

Erysipelas

• Soak 1 kg whole wheat in 1,500 ml water for 3 days; crush the wheat to squeeze out the juice; store juice in a container until it settles, discard the clear liquid; dry the sediment in the sun. Fry the dry sediment over low heat until yellowish; grind into powder. Mix the powder with some rice vinegar. Apply externally to the affected region and its surrounding areas prior to eruption; after the eruption, apply only to the surrounding area, leaving the middle open for drainage of the pus.

• Grind 50 g small red beans into powder; add 3 egg whites to make an ointment. Apply externally to the affected region, one to two times a day. This treatment may also be applied to the swelling of carbuncle and burns.

Burn

• A Chinese physician reported, "In the past 20 years, I have applied fresh ginger juice to treat 400 or 500 cases of burns by hot water or fire, and I have not failed a single case." To use his treatment method, crush fresh ginger and squeeze out juice. Apply it to burns with a cotton ball, which should stop pain instantly; and it can also heal inflammation, reduce swelling, and eliminate blisters after the burns have pustulated.
• Apply fresh aloe juice to the burn.
• Crush fresh pumpkin pulp and apply externally to the burn.
• Crush the pulp of fresh wax gourd and apply externally to the burn.

Frostbite

• Chop and crush 5 red chilies; boiling in 100 ml water. Wash the frostbite twice a day.
• Mix 70 ml honey with 30 ml lard to make an ointment. Apply externally to the frostbite.
• Heat chilies in sesame oil. Apply the cold oil to the frostbite.
• Soak red chilies in alcohol. Use a cotton ball to apply to the affected region, 3 times a day, both for a cure and to prevent future attacks.

Vitiligo

• Slice a piece of fresh ginger or garlic clove. Rub the affected region until the juice is gone; repeat the same procedure with a new slice of ginger or garlic until hot sensations are generated in the skin, 3 to 4 times a day, until the skin returns to normal. This treatment may also be applied to alopecia areata and alopecia prematura.

Alopecia Areata and Alopecia Prematura

• Cook sesame seeds until half burned; grind into powder and mix with cold lard to make an ointment. Apply externally to the affected region, a few times daily, until hair starts growing again.
• Cut up and crush 10 g red chilies; soak in 50 ml white wine (60 percent alcohol) for 10 days; strain and apply the wine to the affected region, a few times daily.
• Treat the same way as vitiligo.

Fungus Infection, Scald, Tinea Corporis and Psoriasis

• Cut up and crush 250 g fresh ginger and soak it in 500 ml white wine for 2 days. Use a cotton ball to apply externally to the affected region, several times a day.

• Crush peeled garlic cloves; mix with sesame oil or lard to make an ointment. Cut the hair in the affected area before application, once a day, and apply externally to the affected region.

• Mix 20 g whole cloves with 70 percent alcohol to make 100 ml. Apply externally to the affected region.

• Apply vinegar to the affected region, 3 times a day. Or fill a plastic bag with vinegar and tie the bag around the hand overnight to heal greyish nails.

• Boil a few eggs and remove the egg white; fry the yolks until dried and burned; mix yolks with boiling water so that yolk oil will float on the surface. Cool it and use to rub the affected region.

Insomnia

• Crush an onion and put it in a jar. Inhale the vapor through the nose while in bed. Normally you fall asleep within 15 minutes.

• Wrap 30 g wheat bran in a clean cloth as a tea bag; make tea with the bran. Drink it all at once before bedtime.

• Prepare 50 g fresh lily flowers (reduced by half if dried lily flowers are used) and 15 g rock sugar; boil in water for 30 minutes; remove the lily flowers; add 15 g rock sugar to the liquid and boil for 2 minutes. Drink 1 hour before bedtime, once a day for 1 week.

• Eat cooked egg yolk every day for a few weeks.

• Fry 20 g wheat until yellowish; add 5 g licorice and 10 red dates; boil the 3 ingredients in water over low heat until water is reduced by half. Drink as soup.

Neurasthenia

• See the last remedy under Insomnia.

• Regular consumption of honey with milk at breakfast is a good remedy.

• Regularly eat garlic.

• Regularly eat walnuts.

Hiccupping

• A Chinese physician in the Hebei Provincial Hospital in China reports he has cured more than 30 cases of hiccupping with fresh ginger slices. But he cautions that when the patient under treatment is also suffering from acute mouth infections or laryngitis, this method should be applied with great care. The method is as follows: Select juicy fresh ginger and cut it in slices; when hiccupping occurs, put 1 ginger slice in the mouth and chew it slowly and swallow the juice; in general, 1 to 3 slices should stop the hiccupping.

• Boil 15 g sword beans in water. Drink it as soup.

• Bake fresh litchis with shells until half charred; grind into powder. Drink with warm water.

• Prepare 30 g fresh ginger and squeeze out the juice; mix with 30 ml honey. Slowly drink it all.

• Mix 20 ml rice vinegar with an equal amount of cold water. Slowly drink it all.

Chronic Constipation

• Peel and chop 500 g sweet potatoes as you would in normal cooking: boil the potatoes in water; add salt or sugar as seasoning. Eat before bedtime.

• Cut up 100 g white radish and squeeze out the juice; mix with some honey. Eat every day.

• Mix 2 teaspoonfuls honey with a glass warm water. Drink it on an empty stomach first thing in the morning.

• Cut up and crush fresh unpeeled potatoes and squeeze out the juice. Drink 2 teaspoonfuls of the juice with honey on an empty stomach first thing in the morning for 2 to 3 weeks. This remedy also applies to gastric and duodenal ulcers.

• Crush 7 star anise, 20 g hemp, and 7 green onion white heads; boil in water. Eat it twice a day. This also applies to difficulty when urinating.

• Eat a few very ripe bananas or dry figs on an empty stomach first thing in the morning (hard bananas could produce negative results).

• Regularly drink milk first thing in the morning on an empty stomach.

• Soak 1 glass rice in water overnight. Next day, boil 10 walnuts for 5 minutes; grind them in a blender; pour the rice and soaking water into the blender and grind them again; add more water and a little sugar and continue boiling the walnuts and rice over low heat until they become sticky. Eat this dish regularly.

• Drink a glass grapefruit juice first thing in the morning on an empty stomach.

Enuresis and Frequent Urination

• Chew a few fresh chestnuts (uncooked) in the morning and in the evening to reduce frequent urination, particularly in older persons.

• Mix half a spoonful of ground cinnamon twig with maltose and a little licorice powder. Drink twice a day to stop bed-wetting in children.

• Soak 30 dried mushrooms in water until they are soft; cook with a few green onion white heads, add soy sauce as seasoning, for normal consumption at meals.

• Steam 2 chicken livers with 3 g ground cinnamon and a little water. Eat the livers to relieve frequent urination and enuresis in children. This cannot be taken by pregnant women, for cinnamon is very pungent and hot, which could cause damage to the energy of the fetus.

• Boil 150 g string beans in water; add a little salt as seasoning when the beans become very soft. Drink as soup on an empty stomach to stop frequent urination.

Diarrhea

• A Chinese hospital in Shanghai presents this simple remedy effective for the treatment of diarrhea: Peel 2 cloves garlic (about 15 g) and crush them; add 2 teaspoonfuls brown sugar, and boil the 2 ingredients in half a glass water. Drink the hot soup each time, 2 to 3 times daily.

• Eat 1 peeled crabapple first thing in the morning on an empty stomach; eat a crabapple after lunch and another after dinner.

• Fry fresh ginger without oil until it becomes dry and burned on the outside; grind into powder. Take 8 g ground ginger each time, 3 times a day, with warm water.

• Crush a few fresh radishes to squeeze out the juice. Drink a cup of juice each time, twice a day.

• Boil in water 60 g fried hyacinth beans with 60 g yam and 50 g white long-grain rice (not brown rice). Drink it as soup.

• Boil a chicken egg until hard cooked; peel the shell and save the egg white for another dish; place the yolk in a fry pan to fry over low heat to extract the oil. The oil of 1 egg may be used as a one-day dosage for infants under a year old, divided into 3 dosages; children over one year may take the oil of 2 eggs in 1 day; each treatment program lasts 4 to 5 days. This recipe is particularly designed for diarrhea or vomiting in infants due to simple indigestion; it is not good for chronic indigestion or diarrhea. In general, improvement in stools should appear in 2 to 3 days; otherwise, stop the treatment.

• Fry 3 bean curds in peanut oil over low heat; add a little salt and 60 ml rice vinegar and boil for a short while. Eat it for relief of diarrhea.

• Bring a glass of water to a boil; crack a duck egg into the boiling water and stir it; add 1 teaspoonful fresh ginger juice and a little salt as seasoning. Eat the bean curds and drink the soup.

Hoarseness

• Crush a few pears and squeeze out the juice. Drink it slowly.
• Boil 50 fresh peanuts in water. Eat every day.
• Mix a teaspoonful of honey with a glass of warm water. Drink it 3 hours after meals, 3 times a day for 1 week. This is beneficial to sudden loss of voice or hoarseness due to excessive fatigue, but not beneficial to loss of voice in common cold.

Coughing

• Slice 2 snow pears into small pieces; add 3 bowls water and boil until the water is reduced to 2 bowls; strain and discard the pears; add 30 g white rice to the liquid and boil again until cooked. Drink the rice soup.
• Peel 200 g fresh radishes and cut into small pieces; prepare 1 or 2 gold carps by removing the internal organs without scraping off the scales; simmer the radishes and carps and add some seasoning. Drink the soup.
• Peel 50 g fresh ginger and cut into small slices; boil the ginger slices with 100 g maltose in 2 glasses water for 30 minutes. Drink it hot, twice a day, in 1 day.
• Boil 20 red dates with 60 g maltose in an adequate amount of water. Eat once a day.
• Mix 150 ml fresh lotus juice with 30 g honey. Drink as juice, once a day, for a few days.
• Make a hole on the side of a pear or an apple; pour some honey into the hole; steam the pear or the apple. Crush it and eat.

Edema

• Use 15 g of the shells of dried broad beans and 6 g red tea leaves to make tea or to simmer over low heat. Drink the juice regularly.
• Remove and discard the internal organs of a chicken; squeeze 60 g small red beans into the chicken cavity; simmer in water and season the chicken. Eat the chicken and beans and drink the broth.
• Boil 60 g mung beans in water with 100 g pork liver and an adequate amount of white rice. Season and eat the stew.
• Boil 60 g Job's tears in water with an adequate amount of white rice. Season the soup before eating it.

Vomiting

• Three Chinese physicians report they jointly treated 20 cases of vomiting with remarkable results. To use their remedy, first, fry 20 to 30 g long-grain rice until yellowish; second, cut up some fresh ginger, add a little salt, then wrap them in a wet paper towel and heat in a pan; third, prepare 30 g honey; fourth, fry 1 to 2 g salt on high heat. After the above ingredients are ready, boil the yellowish rice in 1 cup water until rice breaks to look like flowers. Add the ginger, salt, and honey. Let the patient take 3 to 5 teaspoonfuls of this remedy at first, and then continue to take more very slowly, about 10 minutes later; in general, vomiting should stop in half an hour.

• Steam 2 teaspoonfuls fresh chive juice with 1 teaspoonful fresh ginger juice and 250 ml fresh milk. Drink it warm before meals.

• See the remedies under Hiccupping.

• Chew a few preserved plums slowly, like chewing gum.

• Grate 50 g fresh ginger and make tea with 100 g dried orange peel and water; drink it slowly. This is particularly recommended for people who develop the urge to vomit at the sight of foods.

• In case of dry vomiting, mix a teaspoonful of honey with a small cup fresh ginger juice. Drink it slowly.

• For chronic vomiting with cold sensations, prepare 7 black dates and a few whole cloves; crush the cloves and boil with the dates in water. Eat the dates and drink the soup on an empty stomach, once a day for 1 week, as a treatment program.

Nosebleed

• A Chinese physician writes, "In recent years, I have been treating cases of persisting nosebleed with a simple remedy and achieved instant results usually with a single treatment. Prepare a fresh tender onion leaf and cut it open, use a cotton ball to rub the inner surface of the onion leaf until the cotton ball becomes soaked with onion fluids; squeeze the cotton ball into the bleeding nose, which should stop the bleeding. This method is effective for nosebleed of various causes."

• Wash fresh lotus roots with cold water; peel and crush them to squeeze out the juice. Drink 2 cups a day; this recipe is also a good remedy for coughing up blood resulting from pulmonary tuberculosis.

• Crush a few garlic cloves and make a cake. Place it in the sole of the foot as an external treatment.

• Squeeze the juice out of fresh chives. Drink a small cup of juice each time, twice a day.

11

Chinese Diet For Weight Loss

THE CHINESE THEORY OF OVERWEIGHT

Any useful or scientific theory should be based upon facts; otherwise, the theory is sheer speculation. But what are the facts?

It is a fact that Chinese emigrants do not become overweight as easily as their children born in the West. This phenomenon is obvious in Hawaii where there are as many overweight Orientals as Caucasians, which allows us to reason that obesity has no racial discrimination. In other words, anyone—Oriental or Caucasian—born in the West has an equal opportunity to become overweight. But I have not met any Oriental immigrant who gained more than ten pounds after coming to the West. I have seen many immigrants gain eight pounds during the first year after their arrival. But their weight normally declined again within a year to maintain more or less the same as their weight in the Orient. A dramatic change in their diets caused the initial weight gain. Of course, a small number of Chinese immigrants remain overweight because they were overweight before they emigrated.

Since a person's native country should not influence his or her weight, I believe overweight in later life is already determined when a person has reached ten years of age. Similar to the theory in psychology that personality is already determined before ten years of age (or even earlier), I believe this concept is applicable also to obesity. Undoubtedly, some people have a greater tendency to become overweight due to hereditary factors; heredity plays a role in psychology and physiology. The crucial factors, however, are not the hereditary (predetermined) factors, but the environmental ones that may be altered and influenced. This does not mean that after age ten, a person will remain overweight or underweight, no matter what he or she eats or does; it only means that after age ten, an obese person will be heading in the direction of obesity and that a nonobese person will be moving away from obesity unless something is done to change the direction.

HEADING TOWARDS OBESITY OR SLENDERNESS

What makes one person bound for obesity and another for slenderness? The growth of the human body may be compared to that of a tree. When the tree foundations are solidly built, the tree will be strong and more difficult to destroy at a later stage. In a similar way, when a person's internal organs are solidly built at an early age, the person will be strong and it will be more difficult to later weaken him or her. In other words, when the internal organs are nourished well in childhood, they tend to work hard afterwards and make you overweight; this is why the Chinese immigrants in the West do not become overweight easily; their internal organs were not overnourished when they were young.

There are always two factors at work when considerating obesity: What you are and what you eat. Some people eat a lot but remain skinny; others eat a little but become overweight. I remember having a conversation with an excessively overweight gentleman in my Vancouver clinic who told me he was taking vitamins as food supplements every day. I saw no reason why it was necessary for him to take vitamins, particularly when he was so heavy. But this gentleman emphatically replied, "I do not believe vitamins will put on weight, do you?" The question is, do vitamins contribute to obesity?

If you think that only one factor (the foods you eat) contribute to obesity, it is obvious that vitamins have nothing to do with obesity; modern knowledge of vitamins indicates they will not contribute to obesity. But if you realize there are *two* factors contributing to obesity (what you are and what you eat), then you know that vitamins may contribute to obesity. If they are worth anything at all, vitamins must contribute to the body in a positive manner. For example, vitamin B-1 can increase appetite and absorption and vitamin D can promote normal growth of bone and teeth. This means that vitamins improve the conditions of the body and indirectly contribute to obesity, because when the body conditions are stronger they have a greater capacity to work hard during the digestion and absorption processes.

But it is not my intention to attack vitamins as culprits of obesity; my only purpose here is to point out the two factors that contribute to the problem of obesity and that both factors should be considered. When a person is overnourished at an early age, the internal organs in general, and the digestive system in particular, will develop a far greater capacity for digestion and absorption, which make this person bound for obesity later in life. I deliberately use the word overnourished (as opposed to undernourished) because it indicates something undesirable. Under normal circumstances, we naturally think in terms of "the more, the better." For example, we believe that the stronger our body is, the better, that the more money we have, the better, and that the longer we live, the better. And so, we have a natural tendency to think that the more our body is nourished, the better. This is a crucial error we make in nutrition and human health. It is not always true that the more our body is nourished, the better; we must add another condition to make it a true statement: The more our body is nourished, the better, provided the body is well balanced. A strong, imbalanced body is just as bad as a weak, balanced body.

A WELL-BALANCED BODY

A well-balanced body means that the body is equally in shape in all respects. For example, a person with a strong stomach but a weak heart, or a strong heart but a weak liver, or who is strong and energetic but who suddenly dies of a heart attack is not well-balanced; a person whose internal organs remain in good shape but suffers from hepatitis is not well-balanced.

It is interesting to see that our internal organs are not always cooperative with each other; when a given organ is excessively strong, it will weaken another organ or even cause harm to another organ. It would be nice if all of our internal organs could be equally nourished or even equally over-nourished, because in that case, we would be very strong and live a long, happy life. Unfortunately, this has not happened before and is not happening now, even in this affluent society; on the contrary, far more cases of diabetes, hypertension, cancers, and what not have developed, all of which point to the fact that as it is, our body is overnourished but not balanced. This means that our internal organs are not overnourished equally. We have overnourished our digestive system at the expense of other internal organs, which is why we have more cases of heart, kidney, and liver diseases, which are not directly related to the digestive system.

According to the Chinese theory of internal organs, when the stomach and spleen are overnourished, it weakens the kidneys and bladder; when the kidneys and bladder are overnourished, it weakens the lungs and large intestine; when the lungs and large intestine are overnourished, it weakens the liver and gall bladder; when the liver and the gall bladder are overnourished, it weakens the stomach and spleen. Under normal circumstances, we eat what we like most, and the mouth is the final judge of our preferences, and so, we eat according to our own taste dictated by the tongue or the mouth. But the mouth is only a representative of the stomach; it does not represent other organs, such as the liver or the heart or the lungs.

Ideally, all our internal organs should have equal representation in the mouth to guarantee fairness in the selection of foods, as in a democratic political system in which all regions of the nation should have representation in the central government. Since there is no equal representation of internal organs in the mouth, we eat just to please the mouth and the stomach it represents. Small wonder that we eat only for enjoyment and to put on weight. Sweet foods are pleasing to the mouth, so we eat them most frequently and in large quantities; bitter foods are good for the heart, but we seldom eat them, because they are not pleasing to the mouth; pungent foods are good for the lungs, but we don't eat them as often as sweet foods, because they are not particularly pleasing to the mouth; salty foods are good for the kidneys and gall bladder, but we do not particularly enjoy them, because they are not very pleasing to the mouth; sour foods are good for the liver and gall bladder, but we do not eat them often, because they are not particularly pleasing to the mouth. In short, we eat only to please the mouth and the stomach, which means to enjoy the taste and to gain weight as a result. This used to be good in the past when our stomachs were undernourished due to poverty, but now, in modern affluent society, it becomes bad.

ENJOYING MEALS AND STAYING SLIM

It is not only possible but also realistic to enjoy your meals and stay slim at the same time. There are many possible ways of losing weight, but most are unrealistic and unworkable in real life: For example, losing weight by fasting is possible and effective, but unrealistic and dangerous in practice; losing weight by following those strict diet books is possible and may be effective, but it is not realistic because you eventually get sick of it, and no doubt, you will quit; losing weight by going to weight control and diet clinics is possible and effective, but also unrealistic, because after a while, you will give up and gain back all the weight before you know it. As far as I can see, a realistic and long-term approach to weight loss is to be able to enjoy your meals and lose weight or stay slim at the same time. But can it be done? The answer is emphatically yes.

Expensive foods please our taste and overnourish our stomach, because the mouth (or taste) is a representative of the stomach. There are ways by which foods may be mixed to please the mouth without overnourishing the stomach, however, and this is called the art of cooking. Let us assume that we have three ingredients: the first one is pleasing to the taste, the second is neutral, and the third is repugnant to the taste. The three ingredients may be cooked together in such a way that they become pleasing to the taste, and yet they do not overnourish the stomach. I will give a few examples to demonstrate how this is possible and also realistic.

Chinese meat sauce: This standard recipe for meat sauce has ten ingredients listed below with their energies, flavors, and organic actions:

Dry orange peel—warm; pungent and bitter; affects the spleen and lungs.
Star anise—warm; pungent and sweet; affects the spleen and kidneys.
Cinnamon bark—hot; pungent and sweet; affects the liver and kidneys.
Cloves—warm; pungent; affects the stomach, spleen, and kidneys.
Green onion white heads—warm; pungent; affects the lungs and stomach.
Fennel—warm; pungent; affects the kidneys, bladder, and stomach.
Red chili—hot; pungent; affects the heart and spleen.
Black pepper—hot; pungent; affects the stomach and large intestine.
Nutmeg—warm; pungent; affects the spleen and large intestine.
Licorice—neutral; sweet; affects the lungs, stomach, and spleen.

Wrap the sauce ingredients in a clean cloth; boil in water with wine, soy sauce, and some sugar. After the sauce is ready, the meat can be either soaked in the meat sauce for a few hours or simmered in the sauce for as long as two hours, which should thoroughly mix the meat with the sauce. But meat sauce is not meat soup and it cannot be drunk. The leftover sauce should be used in the next few days, but to preserve it, it is wise to boil the same sauce daily.

As you can see, many of the above ingredients by themselves are not pleasing to the taste at all. For example, few of us will like the taste of cloves or fennel or star anise. But when mixed with meat, they make a delicious dish. Moreover, virtually all internal organs and most flavors and energies are looked after. When this sauce is used to cook meat, the meat will not only be delicious, but will not put on weight because the warm, hot, and pungent ingredients make it very yang. This is why I believe that it is not only possible, but also realistic to enjoy meals and stay slim at the same time.

Soups: Another example is the Chinese habit of making delicious soups— mushroom, chicken, beef, egg, pork, fish, clam soup, and many others. Soups are delicious and will also help you lose weight. I have pointed out that it is the quality of foods not their quantity that really contributes to your gaining weight, but when the same foods are to be consumed, the quality does make a difference. For example, 1 pound of beef (450 g) is certainly different from 100 g, in terms of the effects on weight control. Everything else being equal, eating 1 pound of beef will put on more weight than eating 100 g; and drinking soups will make you consume less foods without sacrificing your enjoyment of good meals. For example, 100 g beef may seem like a very small quantity when it is used for a beefsteak, but when making soup, its quantity is significantly increased.

To make *beef soup*, cut up 100 g beef into small pieces; place in a bowl, add a little wine and five small slices of fresh ginger and an adequate amount of water. Simmer the soup over low heat for an hour. This should make a delicious beef soup. Or, you can steam the ingredients for 2 hours. This beef soup will not put on weight. On the contrary, I believe it will make you lose weight and stay slim, because it will make you eat less as a result. Moreover, this beef soup contains wine and ginger, which act upon many other internal organs, in addition to the stomach, one of the best ways of eating beef without gaining weight. The same principle applies to making other soups to lose weight or stay slim.

How can soups promote good health?

- *Beef soup* is good for weakness and anemia.
- *Chicken soup* is good for fatigue and neurasthenia.
- *Mung bean soup* is good for inflammation of the internal organs.
- *Mushroom soup* is good for weak liver.
- *Clam soup* is good for hypertension.
- *Longevity soup* is made by using bones from chicken and pork legs. The

bones should be crushed to extract the marrow, the essence of the bones, which is considered the most precious part of bone soup. In making the bone soup, soak the bones in the Chinese meat sauce (described above) and then simmer over low heat with other ingredients, such as peanuts, mushrooms, red beans, or radishes, and then season with red chili powder or black pepper.

ELIMINATING FAT IN MEATS

There are external and internal methods of eliminating meat fat. The external methods include cutting and discarding the fat before eating; and the use of meat sauce is partially intended to neutralize the effects of fat in meats. Also, in cooking pork (which contains a higher percentage of fat), boil pork for 20 to 30 minutes; remove the pork and wash it with cold water. This is one way of reducing fat in pork. Some fat will get into our body and something needs to be done about it and this is the internal method of removing or reducing fat in meats.

The Mongol people, who consume more meats than other people, rely on drinking large quantities of strong tea to counteract the effects of fat in meats. In Peking, for instance, customers served Mongolian roast meat are routinely offered a special wine believed to have the strong effect of dissolving the fat in the body; after the meal, a cup of strong tea is served as a way of reducing the effects of fat. As a test, next time you drink tea, don't throw away the tea leaves. Instead, use them to clean some fat from your hands to see how effective tea leaves are in removing grease. Then you can easily imagine the same effects taking place inside your body after you drink tea. Therefore, regular consumption of strong tea is another effective way of losing weight and staying slim. A doctor friend who recently returned from England said he was very surprised to find that the British people generally are much slimmer than their American and Canadian counterparts, which may be attributed to the British habit of tea-drinking.

For weight loss, green is better than black tea, because the effects of black tea are weakened by fermentation. In making tea, the water should be boiling; first, pour a little boiling water to warm up the teapot; then, measure the tea leaves in the teapot and quickly pour the boiling water into the teapot. Wait for a few minutes before drinking the tea. Expensive tea, like expensive foods, is not good for weight loss; the tea should be strong and bitter, which is less expensive. Expensive tea leaves can be used only once, but less expensive tea leaves may be used 2 or 3 times in a day, then discarded.

These broad principles may be generally useful to overweight people, but there are individual physical constitutions that should also be considered for a better solution to the problem of obesity. Two people may eat identical foods in identical quantity, but one may be overweight while the other may be underweight, due to the difference in their physical constitutions.

PHYSICAL CONSTITUTIONS AND OBESITY

Two types of physical constitutions have a tendency to become obese: hot-damp, and cold-damp types. People with hot-dry physical constitutions never become overweight no matter what or how much they eat; as a group, they are practically free of obesity. A rooster is the typical creature with a hot-dry physical constitution. Have you ever seen a fat rooster? I have not. When I was a little boy, I used to feed our chickens (and I always fed them equally without sexual discrimination, because I simply spread the rice on the ground and let them eat; whether roosters or hens was none of my business). I noticed that roosters always ate faster than hens, they were quicker and more aggressive. But to my great disappointment, hens easily became fat whereas roosters always remained skinny. I wished all of them would gain weight fast so that we could sell them and earn lots of money. Now you see, foods alone cannot be responsible for obesity; it is only when certain foods are consumed by certain people that obesity occurs.

The ultimate goal, therefore, is make the physical constitutions of overweight people hot and dry. Overweight people usually have a damp physical constitution; they retain an excessive amount of water in the body, making them overweight.

DEALING WITH OBESITY

Chinese physicians developed four methods of drying the body, a prerequisite in dealing with obesity: The first is to promote urination, which may be compared to diuretics in Western medicine. Small red beans, corn and corn silk, Job's tears, and the peel of wax gourd significantly promote urination.

Small red beans may be eaten often as a food. But it is frequently used in Chinese herbalism as an effective herb to promote urination, particularly in the treatment of edema in nephritis and beriberi. Small red beans look like ordinary red beans but are shaped longer and are more effective. They may be boiled with malt or red dates and a few garlic cloves.

Some people think that the more you eat, the more weight you will gain, which is not true. According to the traditional Chinese theory, it depends on *what* you are eating. The more small red beans you eat, for example, the more weight you will lose. Therefore, small red beans are absolutely not recommended for skinny people, particularly children, because a prolonged consumption of them will make them lose weight. If you look at a standard nutrition book, you read that 100 g small red beans contain 319 calories, which is about the same as beefsteak. There is a basic difference between the two, however, in what the beans and steak can do, not what each of them has. It is true that both small red beans and beefsteak have about 300 calories per 100 g but it is important to remember that small red beans can promote urination and dry up the body, which is lacking in beefsteak.

Job's tears is also used by the Chinese people both as a food and an herb to promote urination. In Chinese herbalism, Job's tears is considered an effective diuretic like small red beans. The Chinese people fry Job's tears, use it to make tea and drink it regularly, particularly when they have difficulty urinating or edema or feel unusually nervous. Job's tears can calm your nerves.

Corn and corn silk are also effective in promoting urination, particularly corn silk, which, according to one experiment, may be used when brewing coffee to promote urination with greater and longer effects.

Soybeans and garlic may also be used to promote urination. Boil 200 g soybeans with 100 g garlic until soft. Eat them at meals. If you don't like garlic, small red beans may be used as a substitute, but garlic is an energy tonic, which can make you feel more energetic, and small red beans have no such effects.

The second method of getting rid of water in the body: Absorb tissue fluids in the body. Absorbing water inside the body is like using a cotton ball to soak up water in a glass; promoting urination removes water from the body through excretion. The majority of foods and herbs that can absorb the water inside the body are aromatic, and the two used most frequently are broad beans and hyacinth beans. The aromatic foods not only can absorb water inside the body, but can stop diarrhea for the same reason. Diarrhea means discharge of extremely watery stools, and when the water is absorbed, the stools dry and there will be no more diarrhea.

Broad beans may be ground into powder to be taken with warm water, but they can also be fried with oil and salt until they break and smell aromatic; use the beans without removing the shell, as the shell has a better effect of absorbing water inside the body and promoting urination.

As for hyacinth beans, use them the same as broad beans. In Chinese herbal therapy, hyacinth beans are very frequently used to relieve diarrhea and abdominal pain due to excessive water in the intestine. They may be used in soup or in powder form.

The third method of eliminating water is to cool the body to facilitate water passage. A dry-hot physical constitution is not prone to obesity as is a damp-hot physical constitution. This is how it works. What happens if you set fire to wet firewood? It won't burn quickly but can only produce smoke, which is bad. Similarly, when water and heat mix in the body, neither will go away. The result is difficulty when urinating or discharge of reddish urine in small quantities. The strategy, therefore, is to cool the body, allowing water to flow. Foods or herbs with a cold energy and a bitter flavor are used for this purpose, because cold energy can cool the body, and bitter flavor can dry it.

Bitter gourd, which tastes extremely bitter, can significantly cool the body, reduce nervous tension due to its cold energy, and also can soften the stools due to its bitter flavor. People with a hot-damp physical constitution often suffer from constipation, which may be effectively relieved by using bitter gourd in soup, as a vegetable, or as tea. Dry or canned bitter gourd may be used as substitutes.

Mung beans, mung bean sprouts or powder may also be used by people with a hot-damp physical constitution to rid the body of excessive water. Although mung bean has a cool energy and a sweet flavor, it is rather effective in removing water and reducing body heat. Mung bean also has an extremely strong detoxicating effect, useful in dealing with many hot symptoms, such as skin eruptions of a hot nature and inflammation of internal organs.

The fourth method of eliminating excessive body water is to warm the body. This method can be used by people with a cold-damp physical constitution, which may be compared to a mountain of ice. The strategy is to warm the body so that the water can flow out of the body, either through urination or perspiration. The foods producing best results should have a warm or hot energy and a pungent-sweet flavor. Hot or warm energy increases body heat, pungent flavor increases perspiration, and a sweet or light flavor promotes urination. Cinnamon twig satisfies these three conditions. A time-honored Chinese herbal formula called five diuretics contains five ingredients: Two absorb water in the body, two promote urination, and the last ingredient, cinnamon twig, is included to warm the body and facilitate water passage.

Regular consumption of fresh ginger can warm the body and induce perspiration simultaneously. Fresh ginger is used frequently to counteract cold particularly in winter, and when it is used along with dry orange peel to make tea, its effects are significantly reinforced.

After the excessive water in the body has been removed and the body is dry, the person should be slim and stay in good shape. But how does a person remain slim and stay in good shape unless the body can stop retaining water?

AVOIDING WATER RETENTION AND STAYING SLIM

An overweight person has two enemies in the body: fat and water. One important thing is to get rid of those enemies and the other is to keep them out of the body. Can and how can this be done? The Chinese believe one thing can do the job and it is called fire.

Many of my students in herbal therapy are at first puzzled by the concept of fire in Chinese medicine. They gradually become used to it, and finally like and appreciate it as a very important and useful concept. Every science consists of concepts and theory; each concept is defined so that it can be used to present a theory. Fire is a concept in Chinese medicine, and a very important one too. What is fire? It is a certain element in the body that functions like fire in cooking. How can fire get rid of fat? By burning it. How can fire get rid of water? By boiling it.

In cooking, fire can burn oil and bring water to a boil so that eventually the water will evaporate. This is a common phenomenon occurring in the human body as well. Is it really nonsensical for the Chinese people to believe that there is fire in the body that keeps burning excessive fat and steaming excessive water out of the body? Is there any fact to prove this is the case? Since I have lots of experiences raising chickens, I'll use them now to prove the point I am making about weight loss.

When you raise chickens for a livelihood as I did when I was a boy, you wish your chickens would quickly grow big and fat to produce a profitable business. But how can you achieve this goal? A hen will grow fat rather easily, but the Chinese people are not very fond of eating hens (their tough flesh is not easy to chew, and their prices are much lower for that reason). On the other hand, a rooster will remain skinny and light as it grows. There is a way to make a rooster grow fat, however, by removing its testis. The rooster will then gain significant weight in a short time, making it even fatter than a hen. This was common knowledge and a common practice shared by all Chinese people when I raised chickens. I certainly did not realize that a few decades later I would use this knowledge about castrated roosters to prove an important point to my Western readers.

The crucial fact is that a castrated rooster is about twice as heavy as a rooster not castrated, and the extra weight is put on soon after castration. Each rooster has one testis, but the presence of this testis in a rooster is crucial in weight control. We all know that in humans and in animals testes are responsible for sexual functions. Men cannot perform sex without testes. But how do the testes contribute to weight loss? In a man the testes heat the body as a heater heats a room. The Chinese physician calls this action the burning fire of the kidneys.

The testes, therefore, are the burning fire of the kidneys. Chinese physicians differentiate between internal (the two kidneys inside the body) and external kidneys (the two testes outside the body). Since women lack testes and their ovaries do not burn as violently as men's testes, small wonder there are more overweight women than men and that it is far easier for women to put on weight than men.

Everything may be classified into yin and yang, including the kidneys. There is kidney yin and kidney yang; kidney yin refers to water in the kidney while kidney yang refers to fire in the kidney. The concept of fire is a very important one in Chinese medicine as mentioned earlier, but what is meant by "kidney fire"? It refers to the kidney's capacity to become energetic, active both in lifestyle and sexual performances. Therefore, in Chinese medicine, when a man becomes sexually impotent, it is attributed to "insufficient kidney fire"; when a man is sexually overactive, it is attributed to "excessive kidney fire".

When a man has a higher level of the burning fire of kidneys, he remains skinny and has a strong sexual capacity. To be slim is to be sexy. A fat fellow will not have a strong sexual capacity, and a fellow with a strong sexual capacity will not be fat; nature does not mix sex with obesity. The burning fire of kidneys will keep burning fat and steaming water out of the body, keeping the body free of obesity. To remain slim and in good shape means you should increase the burning fire of the kidneys.

INCREASING THE BURNING FIRE OF THE KIDNEYS

When I suggest to patients in my clinic that they try to increase the burning fire of their kidneys to lose weight, many jokingly ask me if they need an additional testis to lose weight more effectively. In fact, if this could be done, I imagine it would work in weight control; if someone wishes to lose weight, an extra testis is needed, and to gain weight, one of the testes should be removed. I am amazed that our surgeons, so capable in cutting up the body, have not contemplated the possibility of testes transplantation, which should cure obesity and impotence at the same time and make the medical profession far more respectable. Some people think obesity and impotence are making a mockery of medical doctors as many obese and impotent patients are turned away every day as incurable by our doctors.

Foods called yang tonics can increase the burning fire of kidneys. In Chinese medicine, there are four basic tonics: energy tonics, blood tonics, yin tonics, and yang tonics. A tonic is something that strengthens, and energy tonic refers to something that strengthens the energy, blood tonic to something that strengthens the blood, yin tonic to something that strengthens the fluids, yang tonic to something that strengthens the burning fire of kidneys, also called yang energy in the body. In some cases, different kinds of tonics are used interchangeably, either because a certain food simultaneously performs two or more functions or because one food may be used as a substitute for another.

Animals' kidneys are highly recommended yang tonics, based on the traditional Chinese belief that when human internal organs are weakening, it is beneficial to eat the animal's corresponding organs. Thus, when your liver is weak, you should eat animal liver; when kidneys are weak, eat animal kidneys, and so forth. At a lecture, I remember a lady half-jokingly asked me whether it is beneficial to eat animal's testes or penis when one suffers from impotence. My answer was emphatically yes, which was not a joke. As a matter of fact, when Chinese women with no physiological defects are unable to conceive, they eat animal testes cooked in rice wine (particularly pork testes, which are readily available). And when a Chinese woman consults a Chinese herbalist for infertility or a man for impotence, it is customary for the herbalist to present her or him with the following recipe: Prepare 2 lamb, pork, or beef testes, four kidneys, and 50 g black dates; stir them in rice wine until thoroughly soaked; then steam them. Place the steamed ingredients in a bottle of wine and store for three months before it is ready to drink. This is called yang tonic wine.

Eating kidneys (pork, beef, lamb, or chicken) has three advantages: kidneys have little fat, are easily digested, and tone up the kidney functions. For people who don't like eating kidneys because of their taste, the flavor may be improved. First, cut the kidney in half, remove all unwanted parts and wash it; bring water to a boil and add a little wine; drop in the kidney and simmer until fully cooked; drain and slice into small pieces. Prepare a sauce with ginger, green onion, green pepper, soy sauce, sugar, sesame oil, and vinegar. Pour the sauce over the kidney and it is ready to eat.

Another way to cook kidneys: Cut the kidney in large slices; put 1 tablespoonful oil in a wok or fry pan and as soon as the pan is hot, add sliced ginger, garlic, and chive; stir-fry with the kidney for a few minutes. Garlic, ginger, and chive are condiments and also yang tonics.

For treating impotence in men and frigidity in women, there is another Chinese recipe: cut 2 or 3 garlic cloves into small pieces; fry with 30 g fresh ginger. In fact, if you wish to lose weight and stay slim, use ginger and garlic on a regular basis.

Liver (chicken, pork, and beef) is the second food recommended as a yang tonic to increase the burning fire of the kidneys. Liver can also be cooked to make it pleasing to the taste. Fry the liver very quickly in vegetable oil with condiments, such as ginger, garlic, or celery; use black pepper and wine as seasonings.

Shrimps are the third food recommended as a yang tonic. A celebrated Chinese herbalist in the 16th century advised husbands not to eat shrimps on a journey, intended as a humorous remark to imply that shrimps can dramatically increase sexual desires and they may find themselves in desperation without a sexual partner when separated from their wives. Of course, this advice may not be valid today, because social environments have changed in the course of the past four centuries. Some Chinese herbalists believe that if one consumes too much shrimp without sexual intercourse, one may develop nosebleed due to excessive fire built up in the body.

Shrimps have the greatest capacity for reproduction, it is believed because one single sexual intercourse will produce thousands of eggs, far beyond the human capacity. There are different ways to eat shrimps. Try this traditional Chinese recipe called intoxicated shrimps. Wash the live shrimps and put them in a pan; pour in brandy or whisky, enough to cover the whole shrimps; then add some favorite seasonings, such as ginger, garlic, and sesame oil. Immediately cover the pan because the shrimps will jump like crazy. When the shrimps calm down after a few minutes they are ready to eat. Shrimps may also be fried with garlic to make a strong yang tonic. The Chinese are particularly interested in shrimp's brain (which appears yellowish), shrimp's testes (located on the back), shrimp's liver (turns red immediately on cooking), and shrimp's eggs. The tiny black intestine on the back of the shrimp should be removed before cooking. If fresh shrimps are not available, dried shrimps may be used and cooked with other foods more as a condiment than as a main ingredient.

Mussel is also considered as an effective yang tonic. Mussel has a warm energy, unlike clam (sea or river clam), which has a cold energy. Mussel is a yang tonic; clam is a yin tonic. A Chinese diet classic says, "Cooked mussel can promote erection and heal lumbago." In fact, erection difficulty and lumbago are, in many cases, attributed to weakness of the kidneys, and since mussel is a yang tonic, it should be beneficial to erection difficulty and lumbago. It is believed that mussel can raise body temperature, particularly in the genitals, which is why it is beneficial to sexual impotence in men and frigidity in women.

In China, many women cook mussel with rice wine, ginger, and black soybeans to regulate menstrual flow, because irregular menstrual flow is often caused by coldness in the womb, and mussel cooked with wine can significantly raise womb temperature. The same recipe may be used to warm the genital areas in men. In fact, dried mussel is an important food in Chinese medicine and is normally ground into powder for oral administration. When using dried mussel, wash off the salt, fry and grind the mussel into powder, take 10 g mussel powder with warm water or brandy each time, twice a day, to correct impotence and increase sexual capacity.

In addition to the above yang tonics from animals, the following fruits and vegetables may also be used as yang tonics, including raspberry (it must be dried green raspberry). In China, when summer begins, children pick green raspberries to be used as herbs. They clean the raspberries and soak them in boiling water for 1 to 2 minutes, and then spread them on the ground to dry under the hot sun.

Raspberries can produce effects similar to those of a female hormone, according to an experiment on rabbits and rats. (A Chinese herbalist many centuries ago cautioned men that if they have excessively strong erections that last too long, they should stay away from raspberries.) Like mussel, raspberry can raise the body temperature, particularly in the genitals, and for that reason, is beneficial to women who are unable to conceive due to coldness of the womb. Chinese people also believed that a prolonged consumption of raspberries can improve a woman's skin conditions and prevent hair from graying.

Other foods used as yang tonics include yam (which also acts on the kidneys and stops seminal emission in men and vaginal discharge in women, and it stops frequent urination in both sexes); walnut (which tones up the kidneys and benefits the lungs), chive seed and bitter gourd seed (both good for a wide variety of purposes, particularly in relation to sexual weakness).

If my clinical experiences have taught me anything, it is that a large number of overweight people are not so much interested in a theory of obesity as in losing weight. Many of them ask me, "Can you simply tell me what foods to eat to lost weight?" For this reason I offer a simple and practical answer to the question in the form of a chart, Appendix A. To make use of this chart, determine your own type of physical constitution (as outlined in Chapter 3) and select foods that are good and avoid the foods that are bad for your type; as for foods listed as neutral, eat them whenever you please.

Appendix A

Y-Scores of Foods and Movements of Foods
in Relation to the Seasons

(Foods without indications of y-scores are still undetermined in movements in relation to the seasons.)

FOOD	YANG Outward (Summer)				YANG Upwards (Spring)				Neutral	YIN Downwards (Autumn)				YIN Inward (Winter)			
	+8	+7	+6	+5	+4	+3	+2	+1	0	−1	−2	−3	−4	−5	−6	−7	−8
abalone										x							
apple											x						
apricot									x								
apricot seed (bitter)						x											
apricot seed (sweet)							x										
asparagus							x										
bamboo shoot										x							
banana										x							
barley												x					
bean curd									x								
beef							x										
beetroot							x										
bitter gourd																x	
black and white pepper	x																
black fungus							x										
black sesame seed							x										
brown sugar					x												
butter					x												
cabbage (Chinese)							x										
caraway			x														
carp (common)							x										
carp (gold)							x										
carp (grass)					x												
carrot							x										
castor bean						x											
celery										x							
cherry					x												
cherry seed									x								
chestnut					x												
chicken					x												
chicken egg							x										
chicken egg white												x					
chicken egg yolk							x										
chicory																	
Chinese wax gourd									x								
chive			x														
chive roots			x														
chive seeds						x											

Column groups: **YANG** — Outward (Summer): +8 +7 +6 +5; Upwards (Spring): +4 +3 +2 +1. **Y‑Scores** — Neutral: 0. **YIN** — Downwards (Autumn): −1 −2 −3 −4; Inward (Winter): −5 −6 −7 −8.

FOOD	+8	+7	+6	+5	+4	+3	+2	+1	0	−1	−2	−3	−4	−5	−6	−7	−8
cinnamon bark		x															
cinnamon twig			x														
clam (freshwater)														x			
clam (saltwater)															x		
clamshell (river)														x			
clamshell (sea)															x		
clove			x														
coconut liquid					x												
coconut meat							x										
coconut shell									x								
coffee								x									
common button mushroom									x								
coriander (Chinese parsley)			x														
corn							x										
corn silk							x										
cottonseed	x																
crab																x	
crab apple									x								
cucumber									x								
cuttlebone												x					
cuttlefish													x				
date (red and black)					x												
dillseed			x														
dry mandarin orange peel							x										
duck											x						
eel					x												
eel blood													x				
egg (duck)									x								
eggplant									x								
fennel			x														
fig							x										
fig root																	
garlic			x														
ginger (dried)	x																
ginger (fresh)			x														
ginseng								x									
grape									x								
grapefruit													x				
grapefruit peel						x											
green onion leaf			x														
green onion white head			x														
guava					x												
guava leaf							x										
ham										x							
hawthorn fruit							x										
honey							x										
hops															x		
horse bean (broad bean)							x										

FOOD	YANG Outward (Summer) +8	+7	+6	+5	Upwards (Spring) +4	+3	+2	+1	Neutral 0	YIN Downwards (Autumn) −1	−2	−3	−4	Inward (Winter) −5	−6	−7	−8
hyacinth bean							x										
Job's tears									x								
kelp																x	
kidney (beef)							x										
kidney (pork)												x					
kidney bean							x										
kidney (sheep)					x												
kohlrabi								x									
kumquat						x											
leaf mustard			x														
leek			x														
lemon							x										
lettuce												x					
lettuce (leaf)											x						
lettuce (stalk)																	
licorice							x										
lily flower									x								
litchi							x										
liver (beef)							x										
liver (chicken)					x												
liver (pork)								x									
liver (sheep)												x					
longan					x												
loquat											x						
lotus (fruit, seed, root)							x										
lotus plumule																	x
malt					x												
maltose					x												
mandarin orange											x						
mango											x						
marjoram							x										
milk (cow's)							x										
milk (human)										x							
milk (sheep's)					x												
mung bean									x								
muskmelon											x						
mussel										x							
mutton					x												
nutmeg			x														
olive									x								
onion																	
oyster										x							
oyster shell														x			
papaya							x										
peach							x										
peanut							x										
pear											x						
peppermint							x										
persimmon											x						
pineapple									x								
plum									x								

| | YANG | | Y-Scores | YIN | | | | | | | | | | | | | |
| | Outward (Summer) | | | | Upwards (Spring) | | | Neutral | Downwards (Autumn) | | | | Inward (Winter) | | | |
FOOD	+8	+7	+6	+5	+4	+3	+2	+1	0	−1	−2	−3	−4	−5	−6	−7	−8
polished rice							x										
pork										x							
potato							x										
pumpkir									x								
radish								x									
radish leaf									x								
raspberry							x										
red or green pepper	x																
red small bean									x								
rice bran						x											
rosemary			x														
royal jelly							x										
saffron							x										
salt																x	
sea grass																	x
seaweed																x	
sesame oil									x								
shiitake mushroom							x										
shrimp					x												
sour plum												x					
soybean (black)							x										
soybean (yellow)							x										
soybean oil		x															
spearmint				x													
spinach									x								
squash					x												
star anise				x													
star fruit (carambola)													x				
strawberry											x						
string bean							x										
sugar cane											x						
sunflower seed						x											
sweet basil			x														
sweet potato											x						
sweet rice					x												
sword bean					x												
tangerine orange											x						
taro						x											
taro flower									x								
taro leaf							x										
thyme																	
tobacco			x														
tomato													x				
vinegar										x							
walnut					x												
water chestnut											x						
watermelon											x						
wheat									x								
wheat bran									x								
white fungus							x										
white sugar							x										
wine						x											
yam							x										

Appendix B

Foods in Relation to Energies, Flavors, and Internal Organs

(Foods without indications of y-scores are still undetermined in energies and flavors.)
The symbol " − " indicates "slightly," for example, slightly warm or slightly cold.
The symbol " + " indicates "extremely," for example, extremely sour or extremely cold.

FOOD	Pungent	Sweet	Sour	Bitter	Salty	Cold	Hot	Warm	Cool	Neutral	Lungs	Large Intestine	Small Intestine	Gall Bladder	Bladder	Liver	Kidneys	Spleen	Heart	Stomach	Others
abalone		x			x					x											
apple		x	x						x												
apricot		x	x							x											
apricot seed (bitter)	x			x				x													toxic
apricot seed (sweet)	x			x				x													
asparagus	−x			x					−x												
bamboo shoot		x				x															glossy
banana		x				x															
barley		x			x				x									x		x	
bean curd		x							x		x							x		x	
beef		x						x										x		x	
beetroot		x								x											
bitter gourd				x		x											x	x	x		
black and white pepper	x						x									x				x	
black fungus		x							x		x									x	
black sesame seed		x							x							x	x				
brown sugar		x						x								x		x		x	
butter		x						x													
cabbage (Chinese)		x								x	x									x	glossy
caraway	−x							x									x			x	
carp (common)		x								x						x	x				
carp (gold)		x								x	x							x		x	
carp (grass)		x						x										x		x	
carrot		x								x	x							x			
castor bean	x	x								x	x	x									
celery		x	x							x						x				x	
cherry		x						x													
cherry seed	x		x							x											
chestnut		x						x									x	x		x	
chicken		x						x										x		x	
chicken egg		x								x											
chicken egg white		x							x												
chicken egg yolk		x								x							x		x		
chicory														x		x					
Chinese wax gourd		x							x		x	x	x		x						
chive	x							x								x	x			x	
chive roots	x							x													

179

FOOD	Pungent	Sweet	Sour	Bitter	Salty	Cold	Hot	Warm	Cool	Neutral	Lungs	Large Intestine	Small Intestine	Gall Bladder	Bladder	Liver	Kidneys	Spleen	Heart	Stomach	Others
chive seeds	x			x				x								x	x				
cinnamon bark	x	x					x									x	x	x			
cinnamon twig	x	x						x			x					x			x		
clam (freshwater)		x			x	x										x	x				
clam (saltwater)					x	x														x	
clamshell (river)		x			x	x										x	x				
clamshell (sea)					x	x														x	
clove	x							x								x	x			x	
coconut liquid		−x						x													
coconut meat		x																			obstructive
coconut shell										x											
coffee		x		x				x													
common button mushroom	x								x		x	x	x							x	
coriander (Chinese parsley)	x							x			x							x			
corn		x							x		x									x	
corn silk		x							x					x	x						
cottonseed	x							x													
crab				x		x										x				x	
crab apple		x	x						x		x					x		x			
cucumber		x							x		x						x			x	
cuttlebone					x			−x								x	x				
cuttlefish					x					x						x	x				
date (red and black)		x						x										x		x	
dillseed	x							x									x	x			
dry mandarin orange peel	x			x				x			x							x			
duck		x			x				x		x						x				
eel	x							x								x	x	x			
eel blood	x									x						x	x				
egg (duck)	x					x															
eggplant	x								x			x						x		x	
fennel	x							x								x	x			x	
fig	x								x		x							x			
fig root																					
garlic	x							x			x							x		x	
ginger (dried)	x						x				x							x		x	
ginger (fresh)	x							x			x							x		x	
ginseng		x		−x				x			x							x			
grape		x	x						x		x						x	x			
grapefruit		x	x			x															
grapefruit peel	x	x		x				x						x			x	x			
green onion leaf	x							x													
green onion white head	x							x			x									x	
guava		x						x													obstructive and constrictive
guava leaf		x							x												obstructive
ham					x			x													

FOOD	Pungent	Sweet	Sour	Bitter	Salty	Cold	Hot	Warm	Cool	Neutral	Lungs	Large Intestine	Small Intestine	Gall Bladder	Liver	Kidneys	Spleen	Heart	Stomach	Others
hawthorn fruit	x	x						−x							x		x		x	
honey		x								x	x	x					x			
hops			x					−x												
horse bean (broad bean)		x								x							x		x	
hyacinth bean		x								x							x		x	
Job's tears		x							x		x					x	x			
kelp					x	x												x		
kidney (beef)								x								x				
kidney (pork)					x				x							x				
kidney bean		x							x											
kidney (sheep)		x						x								x				
kohlrabi	x	x		x					x											
kumquat	x	x	x					x												
leaf mustard	x							x			x									
leek	x							x			x				x					obstructive
lemon			+x																	
lettuce		x		x					x		x								x	
lettuce (leaf)		x		x					x		x								x	
lettuce (stalk)																				
licorice		x								x	x						x		x	
lily flower		x							x		x									
litchi		x	x					x							x		x			
liver (beef)		x							x						x					
liver (chicken)		x						−x							x	x				
liver (pork)		x	x					x							x					
liver (sheep)		x	x						x						x					
longan		x						x									x	x		
loquat		x	x						x		x				x		x			
lotus (fruit, seed, root)		x								x						x	x	x		obstructive
lotus plumule				x		x					x					x		x		obstructive
malt		x						−x									x		x	
maltose		x						x			x						x		x	
mandarin orange		x	x						x											
mango		x	x						x											
marjoram	x								x											
milk (cow's)		x								x	x							x	x	
milk (human)		x			x					x	x							x	x	
milk (sheep's)		x						x												
mung bean		x							x									x	x	
muskmelon		x				x												x	x	
mussel					x			x							x	x				
mutton		x						x								x	x			
nutmeg	x							x				x					x			
olive		x	x							x	x								x	obstructive
onion																				
oyster		x			x					x										
oyster shell					x				x						x	x				obstructive
papaya		x								x										
peach		x	x					x												
peanut		x								x	x						x			

FOOD	Pungent	Sweet	Sour	Bitter	Salty	Cold	Hot	Warm	Cool	Neutral	Lungs	Large Intestine	Small Intestine	Gall Bladder	Bladder	Liver	Kidneys	Spleen	Heart	Stomach	Others
pear		x	−x						x		x									x	
peppermint	x								x		x					x					
persimmon		x				x					x	x							x		obstructive
pineapple		x	x							x											
plum		x	x							x						x	x				
polished rice		x								x								x		x	
pork		x			x					x							x	x		x	
potato		x								x											
pumpkin	x			−x																	
radish	x	x							x		x									x	
radish leaf	x			x						x								x		x	
raspberry		x	x					x													
red or green pepper	x						x											x	x		
red small bean		x	x							x			x						x		
rice bran	x	x								x		x								x	
rosemary	x							x													
royal jelly		x																			
saffron		x								x						x			x		
salt					x	x						x	x				x			x	
sea grass				x	x	x															
seaweed					x	x															
sesame oil		x						x													
shiitake mushroom		x								x										x	
shrimp		x						x													
sour plum			+x							x						x					obstructive and constrictive
soybean (black)		x								x							x	x			
soybean (yellow)		x								x	x							x			
soybean oil	x	x						x													
spearmint	x	x						x													
spinach		x							x		x	x									glossy
squash		x						x										x		x	
star anise	x	x						x								x	x	x			
star fruit (carambola)		x	x			x															
strawberry		x	x					x													
string bean		x								x							x	x			
sugar cane		x				x					x									x	
sunflower seed		x						x	x												
sweet basil	x							x			x							x		x	
sweet potato		x								x											
sweet rice		x						x			x									x	
sword bean		x						x				x								x	
tangerine orange		x	x						x									x		x	
taro	x	x								x		x								x	glossy
taro flower										x											numbing taste
taro leaf	x							x													
thyme																					
tobacco	x							x													
tomato		x	x			−x															

FOOD	Pungent	Sweet	Sour	Bitter	Salty	Cold	Hot	Warm	Cool	Neutral	Lungs	Large Intestine	Small Intestine	Gall Bladder	Bladder	Liver	Kidneys	Spleen	Heart	Stomach	Others
vinegar			x	x				x								x				x	
walnut		x						x			x						x				
water chestnut		x				x					x									x	
watermelon		x				x									x				x	x	
wheat		x							x							x	x	x			
wheat bran		x							x											x	
white fungus		x								x											glossy
white sugar		x								x								x			
wine	x	x		x				x			x					x				x	
yam		x								x	x						x	x			

BIBLIOGRAPHY*

Chinese Medical Journal (monthly). Peking, 1959–1984.

Chinese Scientific Nutritional Research Institute. *Nutritional Chart of Chinese Foods*, Peking: People's Health Press, 1963.

Dai Yin-Fong and Liu Cheng-Jun. *Medicinal Uses of Fruits.* Peking: Guang-Xi People's Press, 1982.

Jiangsu New Medical College. *A Complete Dictionary of Chinese Herbs.* Shanghai: Shanghai Technical Press, 1977.

Journal of New Chinese Medicine (monthly). Canton, 1956–1985.

Li Shih-Chen. *An Outline of Materia Medica,* 1578.

Li Yan. *Self Healing of Cancers and Tumors by Herbs and Diet.* Peking: People's Health Press, 1982.

Luo He-Sheng. *Common Herbs for Prevention and Cure of Cancers and Tumors.* Canton: Canton Technical Press, 1981.

Sun Shu Mao. *One Thousand Ounces of Gold Classic,* seventh century. A.D.

Yeh Ju-Quan. *Chinese Diet and Herbal Formulas.* Hong Kong: Shang-Wu Press, 1978.

Yellow Emperor's Classic of Internal Medicine, third century B.C.

*These publications were all published in China in the Chinese language.

INDEX

circulation, 26; of
digestion, 26; of energy
circulation, 26; of milk
secretion, 26; of
urination, 26–27
psoriasis, cure for, 119, 156
pulmonary abscess,
treatment, 101, 102
pulmonary tuberculosis,
cures for, 51–52, 124,
130, 136
pulse: black pepper and, 56
pumpkin, 96–97
pungent foods, 14, 15, 16
purpura hemorrhagica,
cures for, 124
quickening, 119
radish, 97
radish leaf, 97
radix bupleuri, 21
raisins, 65, 66
raspberry, 78; yang tonic,
173
red beans, 107–108
red ginseng, 60
red pepper, 14
respiratory infections, 132
restoring body balance, 32–
34
rheumatic pain, 33:
contraindications, 50
rheumatism cures: carp,
123; fruits, 65–66, 73;
grains, 112–113; spices
and herbs, 54; wine, 133
rheumatoid arthritis, cures,
130
rhizoma cimicifugae, 21
rice bran, 8, 110
rice: sweet (glutinous), 110;
polished (white), 110
rice vinegar, 10–11
rice wine, 10, 133
rickets: cures for, 121–122;
prevention, 99–100
rock sugar, 135
roots: chive, 91; lotus, 80–
81; upward movement
of, 20. (*see also* specific
root)
rosemary, 60
roundworms, 73, 101, 147.
(*see also* ascariasis; biliary
ascariasis)
royal jelly, 130
saffron, 60
salt, 11, 20, 129
saltwater clam, 124
salty foods, 14, 15, 16, 29
scabies, cure of, 115
scald, treatment of, 156
scar elimination, 63
scrofula, cures for, 98
scrotum: swollen, cures for,
94
scurvy, cures for, 99
sea grass, 7, 127–128, 141
seasons: movement of food
and, 21–22; y-scores
and, 43–45
seaweed, 6, 7, 28, 128, 141

seeds: apricot, 77; caraway,
57; cherry, 63–64; chive,
90–91; dill, 20, 49;
fennel, 47–48; lettuce,
94; lotus, 80–81. (*see also*
specific seeds)
seminal emission, 20;
check, 26;
contraindications, 126;
stopping, 73, 81, 82, 90–
91, 102, 109, 123
sesame oil, 115
sex life dichotomy, 40–41
sexual capacity: burning
fire of kidneys and, 170–
171; improvement, 116,
117
sheep's kidney, 117
sheep's liver, 117
sheep's milk, 117
shell powders: crab, 126
shells: oyster, 125
shiitake mushrooms, 99–
100
shoulder pain, 50–51
shrimp, 126, 172–173
sinusitis cures, 92, 130
skin, cracked, 115, 123
skin disease,
contraindications, 47
skin eruptions, 89, 122:
caused by lacquer, cure
for, 125, 126;
contraindications, 89;
spice and herb cures, 54–
55, 57–58
skinniness (*see*
underweight cures)
sleepiness, cures for (*see*
insomnia cures)
small intestine: foods with
organic action for, 25
small red beans, 167
smoking: neutralization of
effects, 62; quitting of,
150
snow fungus, 94
sore throat cures: chicken
egg and white, 119;
contraindications, 51, 56;
fruits, 64–65, 70, 75, 77,
79; grains, 105–106;
legumes, 107; salt, 129;
spices and herbs, 57–58,
61; vegetables, 93, 97,
102–103
soup recipes, 165
sour foods, 14, 15, 16, 29
soybean oil, 112
soybeans, 141, 168: black,
112; yellow, 111
soy sauce, 112
spasm relief, gastric, 121;
muscular, 133
spearmint, 58–59
spices (*see* specific spices)
spinach, 28, 99
spirits, calming down of,
26
spleen: foods acting on, 25,
29; sweet foods and, 14;

tone up, 27
spring: foods, 45; foods
with upward movement
and, 21; y-score, 43–44
sputum: elimination, 26
squash, 101
star anise, 46–47
star fruit, 79–80
stasis ulcer, 121
stigma, 91–92
stomach, 23; falling of, 20–
21; foods acting on, 29;
foods with organic action
for, 25; sweet foods and,
14–15; tone up, 27
stomach falling, cures for,
20–21
stomach upset, cures for:
milk, 117; nuts, 84–85;
spices and herbs, 52, 53,
55–56, 59; vegetables, 95
stomach weakness:
contraindications, 76, 99;
cures, 78–79; 96, 123
stomachache cures, 145–
146: chicken eggshell,
121; fruits, 72, 73, 74–75,
78; honey, 130; nuts, 82;
seafood, 124, 127; spices
and herbs, 47–48, 57;
vegetables, 97; white
sugar, 135
stomach acidity: excess,
cures for, 122
stomatitis, cures for, 112–
113
stones, kidney and
bladder, 82–83
stools: with blood, cure for,
57, 84, 106, 126; dry, cure
for, 117. (*see also* bowel
movements)
strawberry, 77–78
stress, reduction, 125
string bean, 109
sty, eyelid: cures for, 63–64
sugar, 34; in urine, 138–
139; watermelon, 142;
white, 135
sugar cane, 136
sulfur poisoning, cures for,
111
summer: foods with
outward movement and,
21; y-score, 43–44
sunflower seed, 114
sunstroke cures, 98–99,
100–101, 149
suppuration, prevention of,
120
swallowing: accidental, of
coin, 96; difficulty, relief
of, 74, 89–90, 110, 117,
128
sweet foods, 14–15, 16, 29
sweet potato, 96
swelling cures, 89, 98, 124:
of breast, 97; of
carbuncle, 107. (*see also*
edema cures)
sword bean, 38, 108–109

ABOUT THE AUTHOR

Henry C. Lu received his Ph.D. degree from the University of Alberta, Edmonton, Canada. He taught at the University of Alberta and the University of Calgary between 1968 and 1971 and has practised Chinese medicine since 1972. Dr. Lu now teaches Chinese medicine by correspondence. His students live in many countries, including the United States, Canada, England, Australia, Sweden, Italy, Germany, France, New Zealand, Switzerland, Mexico, and Japan.

The author is best known for his translation of *Yellow Emperor's Classic of Internal Medicine* from Chinese into English. This translation and Dr. Lu's seven other books are listed by the Board of Acupuncture Examiners in the United States as references for people registering for licensing examinations to become acupuncturists.

Dr. Lu lectures extensively in the United States and maintains close contacts with the developments of Chinese medicine in China, Japan, Taiwan, and Hong Kong. He has taken groups of Western doctors to study Chinese medicine in China and Taiwan and has helped many distinguished Western physicians establish themselves as outstanding practitioners of Chinese medicine, including herbalism, acupuncture, and manipulative therapy. In March 1982, as leader of a group of Western acupuncturists, Dr. Lu was honored for his knowledge of Chinese medical philosophy by Professor Zhao at the Canton College of Traditional Chinese Medicine.

He has received many awards from acupuncture organizations in the United States and Europe. Dr. Lu is now also patron of Brisbane College of Traditional Acupuncture and Oriental Medicine in Queensland, Australia, and an honorary professor of the Academy of Science for Traditional Chinese Medicine in Victoria, British Columbia, Canada, and an honorary member of the Acupuncture Association of British Columbia.

Dr. Lu lives in Surrey, British Columbia, with his wife, Janet, their son, Albert, and daughter, Magnus. Correspondence with Dr. Lu should be addressed to: Academy of Oriental Heritage, P.O. Box 8066, Blaine, WA 98230 U.S.A. or P.O. Box 35057, Station E, Vancouver, B.C. V6M 4G1, Canada.